A STUDY OF THE BOVINE TUBERCULOSIS ERADICATION SCHEME

Copies of this paper may be obtained from The Economic and Social Research Institute (Limited Company No. 18269). Registered Office: 4 Burlington Road, Dublin 4.

Price IR£5.50
(Special rate for students IR£2.75)

Professor Robert O'Connor is a Consultant with The Economic and Social Research Institute. The paper has been accepted for publication by the Institute which is not responsible for either the content or the views expressed therein.

A STUDY OF THE BOVINE TUBERCULOSIS ERADICATION SCHEME

ROBERT O'CONNOR

ISBN 0 7070 0091 2

Acknowledgements

I am greatly indebted to the following people for help and guidance in preparing this report, for making available statistics and references and for comments on earlier drafts. Professor D.F. Collins and Professor P.J. Quinn, Department of Veterinary Medicine UCD, Messrs K. Maher and P. Rafter, veterinary practitioners and Messrs P. O'B. Gregan, and L.A. Dolan, Veterinary Officers' Association. Messrs J. Butler, P. Hennessy, J. Noonan, M. Sheridan, L.M. O'Reilly, P. Brennan and B. MacClancy, Department of Agriculture, Mr J. Crilly, MRCVS, ACOT, Mr A. Gillis, Irish Farmers' Association and Mr D. Maguire, *Irish Farmers' Journal*. Mr J.G. Shannon, Department of Agriculture Northern Ireland, Mr W.H.G. Rees, Chief Veterinary Officer Ministry of Agriculture, Fisheries and Food, London and Dr J.J. Scully of the EEC Secretariat.

I am also deeply grateful to Mr T. Baker, Dr E. O'Malley, Mr J. Roughan and Professor K.A. Kennedy of The Economic and Social Research Institute for reading earlier drafts and making valuable suggestions.

Finally, I would like to thank the clerical staff of the ESRI for typing and reproducing all the drafts and Ms M. McElhone for preparing the manuscript for publication. I alone am responsible for the final draft and for any errors or omissions.

CONTENTS

		Page
Acknowledgements		iv
General Summary		1
Introduction		10

Chapter

1   *THE NATURE OF THE DISEASE AND ITS CONTROL*   12

Cross Infection from Cattle to Humans; Eradication Methods; Methods of Eradication using the Tuberculin Test; Maintenance of Herds Free from Tuberculosis; Incidence in Badgers; The Badger Situation in Britain; The Dunnet Report; Incidence in Other Animals; Incentive to Eradication; The Epidemiology of Tuberculosis Contrasted with that of Brucellosis.

2   *HISTORY OF THE BOVINE TUBERCULOSIS SCHEME IN IRELAND*   25

Period 1954-1965; Voluntary Stage; Clearance Stage; Animal Identification Card (Blue Card) Stage; Attested Stage; Progress of the Scheme; Period 1966 to Date; Cost to the Exchequer 1954-1965; Costs 1954-1985; Measurement of Tuberculosis Infection; Herd and Animal Incidence; Incidence of Lesions in Non-Reactor Cattle; Incidence of Lesions in Reactor Cattle; The BTE Scheme in Northern Ireland; Comparison of Costs in the Republic with Those in Northern Ireland.

3   *THE OPERATION OF THE SCHEME IN RECENT YEARS*   41

EEC Involvement; Trading Considerations; The Accelerated Plan; Nomination of Testers; High Risk Areas.

4   *DEFECTS IN THE EXISTING SCHEME*   51

Nomination of Testers; Lack of Commitment by All Concerned; High Volume of Cattle Movement; Illegal Movement; Defective Testing; Transport Vehicles; Collection of Reactors and Cattle Dealer Activities;

Re-Testing of Reactor and Inconclusive Herds; Depopulation of Herds and Additional Funding; Epidemiology; Financial Contribution from the Farming Sector; National Manager and Executive Office; Animal Identification; Disinfection of Premises; Severe Interpretation of the Test.

5   *CONCLUSIONS AND RECOMMENDATIONS*   61

Cattle Movement Contact and Trace Back; Identification of Cattle; Illegal Movement and Other Illegal Practices; Nomination of Testers; Reliability of the Test and Defective Testing; Lack of Commitment to the Scheme by All Concerned; Transport Vehicles; Collection of Reactors; Disinfection of Premises; Financial Contribution from the Farming Sector and Funding of the Scheme Generally; Transferring the Eradication Scheme to an Executive Office under a National Manager; Strategy Plan.

References   74

Appendix

A   *RELIABILITY OF THE TUBERCULIN TEST*   78

B   *REACTOR COMPENSATION, RATES OF GRANT (JUNE, 1986)*   82

C   *THE EPIDEMIOLOGY OF TUBERCULOSIS COMPARED WITH THAT OF BRUCELLOSIS*   83

LIST OF TABLES

Table   *Page*

1   Percentage of Cattle Reacting Positively to the Tuberculin Test in Great Britain and South West England 1961-82   18

2   Position Regarding Bovine Tuberculosis in EC Member States and in the USA in 1985   23

3   TB Incidence on Animal Round Testing and Number of Reactors Removed 1966-1985   29

4   Government Expenditure Each Year on the BTE Scheme 1954/55 to 1965/66 at Current and at Constant 1985 Prices   30

5   Government Expenditure Each Year on BTE Scheme 1966-67 to 1985   32

6   Lesions in Non-Reactor Cattle at Registered Meat Factories Compared with Incidence from Testing 1971-1984   35

7   TB Lesions in Reactor Cattle   36

8   Progress in the Eradication of Bovine Tuberculosis in Northern Ireland 1961 to 1984   38

9   Variable Costs in Connection with the BTE Scheme as Percentage of Cattle and Milk Outputs in the Irish Republic and in Northern Ireland   39

10   Bovine Tuberculosis Herd Incidence by County 1980-1984   49

GENERAL SUMMARY

Because of our small domestic market a high proportion of cattle, beef and dairy products have to be exported. Anything which might interfere with these exports would have serious repercussions for the whole economy. The aim must be to ensure that the quality of our produce is regarded as excellent and towards this end it is imperative that bovine tuberculosis be eradicated as soon as possible.

A scheme for the eradication of bovine tuberculosis in Ireland was inaugurated in 1954. Eleven years later in 1965, after the removal of 830,000 reactors the Minister for Agriculture declared that the whole State was free of the disease. Twenty years later, however, after the removal of a further 620,000 reactors it is estimated that 2½ to 3 per cent of cattle herds are still affected and it has now to be considered if the disease can, in fact, be ever eliminated completely.

This paper discusses the nature of the disease, reviews the operation of the eradication scheme since its inauguration and outlines the exchequer costs to date. It examines the operation of similar schemes in Britain and Northern Ireland where the disease has been fairly successfully eradicated to see if there are any lessons to be learned from these and other countries and it makes recommendations as to how we should proceed from now on in light of past experience and taking account of the frictions which have developed over the years between the various institutions and persons.

Nature of the Disease and its Control

Tuberculosis in each species of animal, including man, is caused by one particular type of tuberculosis bacillus though some species are susceptible to more than one type. For example, the human type can give rise to disease in cattle while the bovine type can give rise to disease in man and many other animals. A Royal Commission in England in 1911 reached the conclusion that tuberculosis in cows was a hazard to human health and stated that measures should be taken to remove the hazard. Similarly, in a study in Denmark in 1945, it was concluded that the amount of tuberculosis in human beings was directly related to the degree of the disease in cattle herds with which they had been in contact.

The public health aspect of the disease has tended to be ignored in Ireland

1

in recent years on the grounds that human tuberculosis is almost eliminated and that with BCG vaccination and pasteurisation of milk there is now little danger of contacting the disease from cattle. These views however are not held in other countries. A recent American study says that farm families and slaughterhouse workers can easily be infected by aerosol contamination because of their close association with cattle and these people can spread the disease to others who have no contact with cattle. A few moments' contact with infected animals is often sufficient to set up the disease in man and other animals.

Eradication Methods

A means of early diagnosis and isolation of infected animals is essential in any scheme for the eradication of bovine tuberculosis for by the time clinical signs become apparent in some animals most of the herd will be infected. At present there is no sound blood or other serum test for diagnosing the disease. The tuberculin (skin test) is the most reliable diagnostic method available, but it is not foolproof. Animals not having the disease will often react to the test (false positives) while some of those with the disease may show no reaction (false negatives). It is therefore a rather blunt instrument but it is the only one we have and it has succeeded in eliminating tuberculosis in all the other countries where the disease has been eradicated. Vaccination of cattle with BCG is not a practical proposition and according to the experts has no place in the eradication of bovine tuberculosis.

In an eradication programme all the animals in a country or area are tested. Those showing a reaction to the disease are removed and slaughtered and testing is continued until two successive tests have revealed no reactors. Herds are again tested in 6 months and afterwards at 12 months or 2 yearly intervals if no reactors are found. But even when a country or area is declared free of the disease annual or biennial testing has to be carried on for many years to maintain the position.

Difficulties in Eradication

Tuberculosis is a very difficult disease to clear up. The infective dose is very low; there is no immunity based on age or sex; there is very often no clinical evidence to alert the herdowner of the presence of the disease; transmission occurs 24 hours a day throughout the year and is accelerated by cattle movement along roads and by contact at marts and across fences. Infection spreads rapidly among poorly fed animals or under stressful conditions. The germs are very resistent to environmental conditions and a wide range of animals may act as a reservoir for infection, e.g., badgers, red deer, dogs, cats and goats. Difficulties in lowering the incidence of infection in

South West England where there is a heavy density of cattle are attributed to badger infection in that area. Some Irish veterinary surgeons claim that this animal is a potent carrier here also, but there is no definite proof as yet that this is so.

The disease has been eliminated in a large number of European countries and in the USA, but there is still fairly high infection in Italy, Greece, Spain, Portugal and Ireland. Eradication, however, was not easily attained in any of the countries which are clear of the disease. In Britain it took 27 years to get the disease down to acceptable levels (less than 0.05 per cent of animals). The time taken in the USA was 50 years but like Ireland there were difficulties in that country with cattle movement in the ranching states and with cross border movement from Mexico. In Northern Ireland it took 22 years to get the animal incidence down to 0.04 per cent. At that stage when biennial, and later triennial, testing was introduced the incidence rose again and annual testing had to be resumed in 1982. In Israel eradication started in 1952 and by 1965 the animal incidence was down to 0.01 per cent. Attention was relaxed at this stage and there was a gradual rise to 0.11 per cent in 1968 and it has not been reduced below that level since then. Testing commenced in New Zealand in 1958 and the disease is still not eradicated in that country.

History of the BTE Scheme in Ireland

The eradication programme in Ireland can be divided into two periods. The first period runs from 1954 when the scheme was initiated up to 1965 when the whole State was declared officially free of the disease by the Minister for Agriculture. The second period runs from 1965 to the present time when there is still a relatively high incidence of the disease in the State.

Net expenditure by the Department of Agriculture on the scheme during the first period (gross payments less salvage realisation on reactors) was £368.8 million at 1985 prices. The cost of the scheme from 1965 to 1985, at 1985 prices, was £361 million and when this is added to the 1954/65 expenditure the total cost to the Irish exchequer comes to £730 million. This is somewhat of an overstatement, however. In 1984 and 1985 disease levies paid by farmers were £5.9 million and £13.0 million respectively, while a further £9.5 million was obtained from the EEC in the period 1978 to 1981. Hence net exchequer cost over the whole period, at 1985 prices, was about £691 million.

The above costs, which are described as direct costs, are minimum figures. They do not include overhead costs which are the salaries of the Departmental staff employed on the scheme (about 1,300) either in Dublin or in the District Offices: as these people were also employed on the brucellosis scheme over the past 20 years or so, it is difficult to allocate their salaries. The total overhead costs, from 1954 to 1985, at 1985 prices, was £256 million, and when this sum is divided in proportion to direct expenditure on the two schemes the administration of the tuberculosis eradication scheme over the period comes to £173 million. Adding this to the direct costs brings the total costs (less farmers' levies and EEC payments) over the period to £864 million, at 1985 prices.

In addition to the known exchequer costs there has also been an unknown loss to the economy from the disease. Each year has seen the slaughter of large numbers of reactors, 50 per cent of which are breeding stock (on average about 15,000 per annum). This puts a serious strain on the expansion of the national cattle herd. Also there is a loss of options due to the disease for greater improvement of the national herd through voluntary culling and through failure to achieve farm plans.

Reasons Put Forward for Failure to Eradicate Bovine Tuberculosis

Numerous reports on the eradication of bovine tuberculosis in Ireland have been prepared over the years. Practically all have given reasons as to why the disease has proved so difficult to eradicate, have referred to defects in the existing scheme and made suggestions for improvement. The more important difficulties and defects are listed below and each is then discussed briefly and commented on.[1]

(1) High volume of cattle movement and contact.
(2) Cattle dealer activities and collection of reactors.
(3) Defective testing.
(4) Nomination of testers.
(5) Tag switching and illegal movement.
(6) Failure to depopulate seriously infected herds.
(7) Stop-go funding policies.
(8) Inadequate management of the scheme by the Department of Agriculture.
(9) Absence of annual targets.

High Volume of Cattle Movement and Contact: Because of our peculiar pastoral system of farming, Ireland has a very high volume of cattle movement and contact between animals from different herds at marts, along roads and laneways, and across fences. Unfortunately cattle movement must continue to go on in this country. Too many people depend on it for their livelihood. The best that can be done is to monitor the movements so that

---

1. Defects referred to in many of the reports have since been remedied and are not referred to here.

when diseased animals are found their contacts can be traced and tested. The Department is in the course of computerising all animal records so that an effective movement permit system can be introduced.

Cattle Dealer Activities and Collection of Reactors: Many cattle dealers and farmers put trading considerations before animal health or disease eradication. Reactors are now collected by dealers and hauliers for delivery to slaughter. Though it is illegal to do so, dealers often keep reactors on their farms until they have a full load for the factory and thus infect healthy animals on the same and neighbouring farms. Also there is no way of ensuring that lorries are disinfected after transport of infected animals. Allowing dealers to collect reactors is an abandonment of official control over the movement of known infected animals and is a practice which should be terminated.

Defective Testing: It is claimed that defective testing has contributed significantly to the lack of progress in eradicating the disease in Ireland. An EEC report in 1981 stated that a large number of reactors were being missed on the round tests but this was disputed by the Department of Agriculture whose officials have stated that the trial carried out by the EEC was unscientific and the results unreliable. In any case checking on the reliability of tests is a most difficult task because of the rapidity with which the disease spreads. However, because of a certain amount of public disquiet the matter should be re-examined by a team of outside experts.

Nomination of Testers: Since the scheme was introduced in 1954, until the end of 1984 each herdowner was allowed to nominate the private veterinary surgeon who would test his cattle. An Interdepartmental study group reporting in 1983 stated that there is ample evidence that this close relationship between the herdowner and the practitioner was damaging to the BTE programme. It resulted in pressure on the practitioner to give a "soft" test and there have been numerous examples of a herdowner transferring his testing to another veterinarian after his normal practitioner had disclosed a reactor in the herd.

Arising out of pressures from various sources, the Department attempted to establish the principle that it (the Department) and not the herdowner would have the right to nominate the private veterinarians to do the testing. This development was opposed by the Veterinary Union and culminated in a strike which lasted for about 7 months. This strike was settled in May 1985 with the Department having gained the right to nominate the testers.

In theory this gives the Department greater powers than heretofore over the testers, but in practice there is little change. Veterinary surgeons continue to test their own clients' cattle and there is nothing the Department can do about it except to take action in the rare cases where veterinary surgeons are found to be doing inadequate work or not doing the testing on time. The only way out of this problem would be to have all the testing done by Departmental veterinarians. Staff could be employed on a part-time capacity to do this and paid on a per test basis at little extra cost to that paid for testing now. There would, of course, be many industrial relations problems involved in recruiting such staff and it would be best to wait and see if the disease can be cleared up without having to resort to this measure. If it is not well on the way to being cleared within the next 3 years the Department or some other body may have no option except to have its own staff take over all the testing and seek such staff wherever they can be found.

Tag Switching and Illegal Movement: Cattle, including calves, cannot legally move to other farms from restricted holdings, and herdowners would normally run grave risks in moving older cattle since their registration cards are in the District Office. Unscrupulous herdowners, however, often move cattle illegally by changing their tags. In the past, tags and corresponding registration cards could be obtained from butchers' premises which were not regularly inspected. These used tags could be re-opened and closed again without breaking.

In an attempt to stamp out this practice the Department has been trying for many years to find a tamper-proof tag. Now it has obtained one which seems to be satisfactory in this regard. Once it has been closed with the tagger it cannot be opened again without breaking. The use of this tag should therefore help to curtail tag switching and hence illegal movement of older cattle.

With calves under 6 weeks of age the position is somewhat different. These animals can be moved without an ear-tag and it is therefore impossible to determine where a batch of calves come from. One way out of this problem would be to require that all calves be tested prior to movement and issued with tags and registration cards. To insist on this procedure for all calves would, however, be unduly restrictive and costly since the test would be negative in practically all cases.

The problem could be dealt with by allowing herdowners to tag their own calves and to insist that no calf be allowed to move to another herd without a numbered ear-tag. All calves could thus be traced back to their herd of origin and there would be a check on movement from restricted herds.

It is suggested that this system be adopted here even though it does mean giving out ear-tags to herdowners who may use them for illegal purposes. If, however, farmers were made accountable for all tags received, and fined heavily for missing tags, the system would be workable.

Depopulation of Herds: Bovine tuberculosis is very much akin to human tuberculosis. It becomes endemic in a herd and very often cannot be got rid of without eliminating the entire herd. In the past, depopulation of herds could create very serious social conditions for dairy farmers; the depopulation grant available up to May 1986 was barely sufficient to restock the farm and left nothing for current income. Ordering depopulation therefore placed a great strain on the Department's inspectors and the local veterinary officers. These officials were usually loathe to order complete depopulation because it would often mean bankruptcy for the herdowner. Hence removal of reactors only was all that was recommended while the disease continued to recur because of the presence of carriers which showed no reaction.

The depopulation grant has now been increased substantially and there should therefore be no hesitation about depopulating herds where there is endemic infection. There are only about 400 such herds in the State.

Stop-Go Funding Policies: A problem with the eradication scheme over the years has been a lack of continuity of funding by the government. When funds are scarce the TB scheme gets a proportional cut the same as most other votes. This means that the programme is at best a holding operation which keeps the disease at its present level but will never eliminate it. A proper eradication policy will require non-stop annual rounds of testing for the next 10 years or so and probably biennial rounds for a further 10 years.

Regular funding of the eradication scheme must, therefore, be available but this can never happen if the State is the residual funder. When money is scarce cuts will take place regardless of government promises. What is needed is a levy on herdowners and statutory matching funds from the government to supplement these. If a law setting forth this funding policy were introduced, stop-go policies would cease and we would be able to appraise the effects of a continuous testing scheme over a period.

It is recommended therefore that the present rates of levy payments on cattle, beef and milk be increased by about 13 per cent and that they be extended to include cattle slaughtered for home consumption by butchers. These would give about 75 per cent of direct costs. If costs increase, the levies should be increased accordingly and if costs decrease, the levies should be reduced and dispensed with entirely when the disease is reduced to some agreed level such as say, 0.5 per cent of herds and 0.05 per cent of animals. A policy of this kind should create an incentive on the part of farmers to eradicate the disease as quickly as possible.

Inadequate Management of Scheme: Serious criticisms of the management of the present BTE scheme have been put forward from time to time by the veterinary profession. In general it is believed that the civil service does not have the flexibility required to handle such a scheme and one report has suggested that the operation of the programme be taken out of the Department and set up as an Executive Office under a national manager.

In favour of this change it can be said that the national manager would be independent of the Minister for Agriculture and could take tough decisions without fear of political consequences. But it is doubtful if a national manager could act in a much tougher manner than the present Departmental manager. He would have his own pressures to deal with — the farmers' associations, the veterinary organisations and the Department of Finance.

It could be argued, of course, that the idea of taking the scheme out of the Department should be given a trial, that things cannot be much worse than they are at present. This suggestion has some appeal until one thinks of the problems and frictions involved in getting the scheme out of the Department. It would probably take years to get everything sorted out and this would give excuses for reductions in funding and for lack of commitment to the scheme in the meantime. Hence it seems that we should stick with what we have and try to improve it. If, however, things do not improve, with full rounds of testing over the next 3 years we will have to try something else. Public opinion will demand new approaches in that case.

Absence of Annual Targets: In the early days of the BTE scheme in the 1950s an overall plan for eradication was made and within this plan annual targets were set in relation to the removal of reactors and reduction in the disease incidence. When the country was declared free of the disease in 1965 the programme was deemed to have been completed and formal plans were no longer considerered to be necessary.

In view of events in the meantime, and the persistence of the disease, it seems that a formal plan is once again necessary in order to chart the route to complete eradication. All the evidence suggests that there is only one real solution — intensive annual rounds of testing. All other suggestions for improving the scheme are only incidental. They are necessary but not sufficient conditions.

A plan setting out a time scale for eradication is therefore essential together with the annual costs needed to achieve a series of targets along the way. Such a strategy will put pressure on the government to enact legislation to provide for a constant level of funding as suggested above and for any other reforms which are deemed to be necessary and feasible. We will also need to have check testing carried out on a random sample basis so as to determine the exact incidence of the disease. At present we do not really know what this incidence is and until this is known it will be impossible to set targets for eradication.

Critical Recommendations

This summary of the scheme shows that there are four critical recommendations.

(1) Annual rounds of testing must go on over the next 10 years without stoppage.

(2) The government must make provision for the availability of the necessary funds and decide who shall provide them. It is suggested that herdowners contribute 75 per cent of the variable costs in the forms of levies and the government the remainder. These contributions to be made statutory.

(3) A plan should be prepared for the operation of the scheme over the next 10 years, setting targets for disease incidence each year and estimating costs. It is estimated that the direct costs for the scheme over the next 3 years should be about £28 million per annum at 1985 prices and attempts should be made not to exceed this amount.

(4) If at the end of 1990 it is found that eradication targets are not being met, the operation of the scheme should be taken out of the Department and set up as an Executive Office or semi-State body. In that case testing should be taken over by the new body using temporary staff recruited on a per test payment basis. Many of these staff would be existing practitioners employed on a temporary basis but no practitioner should be allowed test his own clients' cattle.

INTRODUCTION

Though declining, relative to other sectors, Agriculture is still one of the most important industries in Ireland. In 1984 income arising in that sector amounted to IR£1,474 million or to 13 per cent of the national income, while the numbers employed on farms were 181,000 or 16.5 per cent of the total number at work.

In compiling these figures no account is taken of the activity in industries and services involved in supplying inputs to farming and in processing farm output. If these linkages were taken into account the size of the agricultural sector in 1984 would increase to about 23 per cent of the national income or to IR£2,563 million, while the numbers employed would increase by a further 45,000 to 226,000, or to 20 per cent of the numbers at work. Within Agriculture cattle and dairying account for almost 70 per cent of output so that these two enterprises, including their linkages with the food and other industries, contribute about 11 per cent of the national income, or IR£1,260 million.

Because of our small domestic market a very high proportion of our agricultural produce has to be sold outside the country. Cattle and cattle products go overwhelmingly for export with home consumption taking only about 20 per cent of output disposed of. In addition, 60 per cent of milk output is exported. The total value of live cattle, beef and dairy products exported in 1984 was IR£1,162 million, which was 71 per cent of total agricultural exports while the value added of these exports was about 25 per cent of the value added of total exports.

It is obvious from these figures that anything which might interfere with cattle and milk product exports would have serious repercussions for the whole national economy. The aim must be, therefore, to ensure that the quality of our produce is regarded as excellent and towards this end it is imperative that bovine tuberculosis be eradicated as soon as possible.

A scheme for the eradication of bovine tuberculosis in Ireland was inaugurated in 1954. Eleven years later in 1965, after the removal of 830,000 reactors, the Minister for Agriculture declared that the whole State was cleared of the disease. Twenty years later, however, after the removal of a further 620,000 reactors it is estimated that 2½ to 3 per cent of cattle herds are still infected and it has now to be considered if the disease can, in fact, be ever eliminated completely.

The purpose of this study is to:

1. review in detail the operation of the Bovine Tuberculosis Eradication (BTE) scheme since its inception in 1954, outline the exchequer costs

to date and the sectors to which they have been paid, and pinpoint the problems which have arisen, and the mistakes (if any) which have been made;

2. examine the operation of similar schemes in Britain and Northern Ireland where the disease has been fairly successfully eradicated to see if there are any lessons to be learned from such countries; and

3. make recommendations as to how we should proceed from now on, in light of past experience, and taking account of the frictions which have developed over the years between the various institutions and groups involved.

The report contains five chapters. Chapter 1 describes the nature of the disease, the animals affected by the bovine strain, the way the disease spreads, the method of detection and eradication and the measures required to maintain herds free of the disease. A brief review of the situation in regard to the disease in Britain and other countries is given here also. This is a fairly technical chapter but as will become clear later this type of information is needed by the lay reader in order to understand the issues involved and the difficulties arising in the eradication of the disease. The chapter concludes with a section contrasting the epidemiology of tuberculosis with that of brucellosis.

Chapter 2 gives the history of the bovine tuberculosis eradication schemes in Ireland (south and north of the border). The first section of the chapter explains how the eradication scheme was, and is, organised in the Republic, the progress of the scheme, and the costs involved. The second section of the chapter gives a brief outline of the progress of the scheme in Northern Ireland from its inception in 1949 to date.

Chapter 3 gives a fairly detailed description of the operation of the scheme in the Republic of Ireland in recent years. It outlines the number of people employed on the eradication programmes, EEC involvement in the scheme as well as the recent argument regarding the nomination of testers.

In Chapter 4 defects in the existing scheme are outlined, based on statements made in various reports by interdepartmental committees, the Veterinary profession and the Irish Farmers' Association.

Chapter 5 gives the author's conclusions and recommendations relating to the scheme.

The report concludes with three appendices. Appendix A discusses the reliability of the test as judged by the Department of Agriculture and the academic veterinarians. Appendix B shows the rates of grant for reactor compensation as at June 1986, while Appendix C discusses the Epidemology of Tuberculosis compared with that of Brucellosis.

Chapter 1

THE NATURE OF THE DISEASE AND ITS CONTROL

The origin of Bovine Tuberculosis is not very clear but it undoubtedly existed in the Mediterranean area from the early Christian times. It probably existed long before that but exact records are not available to confirm whether or not the domesticated cattle of Asia were infected (Paterson, 1959). The origin of the bacillus causing the disease, *Mycobacterium* bovis (M. bovis) is equally obscure but it is not unlikely that it evolved from the human type (M. tuberculosis hominis).

Tuberculosis in each species of animal including man is caused by one particular type of the tubercle bacillus, though some species are susceptible to more than one type. For example, the human type gives rise to disease under natural conditions chiefly in man, monkeys, pigs and occasionally parrots; the bovine type to disease in cattle, pigs, horses, man and also deer, badgers, opossums and many other wild animals.

There are many other pathenogic types but a large number of species which are found widely distributed in nature, in butter, water, soil, dung, and on the skin of animals, seldom cause disease.

Cross Infection from Cattle to Humans

For many decades the exact nature of bovine tuberculosis and its relationship to "consumption" in man was a matter of considerable debate. During the eighteenth century, for example, the Germans believed that the disease was related to human syphilis, but in 1882 Robert Koch announced that he had observed and cultured the bacillus responsible for the disease in humans and in 1896 the bacterium was given the name *Mycobacterium tuberculosis* (Collins and Grange, 1983).

By the turn of the century bacteriologists had demonstrated that there were small but definite differences in M. tuberculosis strains from human and bovine sources. These findings misled Koch to claim at the British Congress on Tuberculosis in 1901 that "the human subject is immune against infection with bovine bacilli and is so slightly susceptible that it is not necessary to take any steps to counteract risk of infection". Although a majority of workers at the time disagreed with Koch, his brilliant reputation meant that his erroneous statement had far-reaching effects (Grange, 1982). Indeed some scientists in the field continue to feel that by exonerating cows from all blame in the causation of tuberculosis in man Koch put back the clock of veterinary preventative medicine to a degree far greater than is generally accepted.

The positive end product of the controversy surrounding cross-infection from cattle to humans was the appointment of a Royal Commission to investigate the issue. The Commission was active from 1901 to 1911 and its important reports showed that there were three types of bacilli that caused tuberculosis (human, bovine and avian) as well as some others in nature; that human pulmonary (lung) infection acquired from inhalation of bovine tubercule bacilli from cattle was a definite risk; and that bovine tubercule bacilli present in cows' milk causes non-pulmonary (e.g., alimentary canal) tuberculosis in humans.

The Royal Commission also investigated the use of tuberculosis testing in animals which was later to play a crucial role in the bovine tuberculosis control campaigns. The final conclusion reached by the Commission was that tuberculosis in cows was a hazard to human health and that measures should be taken to minimise this hazard.

The public health aspect tends to be ignored in Ireland in recent years on the grounds that human tuberculosis is practically eliminated and that with BCG vaccination and pasteurisation of milk there is now little danger of contacting the disease from cattle. These views, however, are not held in other countries. There is a genuine fear abroad of contacting the disease from infected animals and food. Roberts (1986) says that farm families and slaughterhouse workers can very easily be affected with tuberculosis by aerosol contamination because of their proximity to cattle. A few moments' contact is sufficient to set up an infection. Also, workers in processing plants are exposed to aerosol contamination when slabs of tubercular meat are slapped on to the counter and when the carcases are cut up. There are also documented cases of wound infections causing TB in butchers and veterinarians.

The only reported epidemiological study with a control group was done by Sigurdson in Denmark in 1945 (Francis, 1958). On the farms with tuberculosis positive herds, the proportion of tuberculosis positive persons increased steadily during childhood, reaching 75 per cent at 15 years of age. In contrast, only 15 per cent of the adolescents on the control farms (farms with tuberculin-negative cattle) became infected with TB. On the basis of this study Sigurdson concluded that the amount of tuberculosis in human beings is directly related to the degree of the disease in herds with which they have been in contact. Furthermore, these infected sources infect other people who may have no contact with cattle. These are sobering findings which should help to dispel some of the complacency towards bovine tuberculosis existing in Ireland. They certainly indicate that the public health aspect of the disease cannot be ignored even though the number of human tuberculosis cases notified each year is now only about 800 compared with 1,150 cases in 1978 and almost 7,000 cases in 1952.[2]

Eradication Methods

One of the difficulties with the tubercule bacillus is that even though the different types have different characteristics they cannot be readily distinguished by microscopic examination. They have, therefore, very often to be identified by cultural or biochemical means and sometimes by the slow method of inoculation into laboratory animals.

At present there is no sound serological method (blood or other serum test) of diagnosing tuberculosis. The absence of such a test is a great drawback for, no matter how skilled a veterinary surgeon may be in diagnosing tuberculosis by clinical means, he cannot readily identify infected animals other than those with progressive generalised tuberculosis or active tuberculosis in a particular site. Hence this type of diagnosis cannot be relied upon to form a major part of an eradication programme since many animals will have become infected before they can be so identified and will be passing on the disease to companions. A means of early diagnosis and isolation of infected animals is essential in any scheme for the eradication of the disease for by the time clinical signs become apparent in some animals most or all of the herd will be infected. The efforts that have been made to identify infected animals by clinical examination have usually been directed towards the protection of the public health by removing animals which may be discharging tubercule bacilli in milk or in other ways affecting milk supplies.

The tuberculin test is the most reliable diagnostic method available for mass use at the moment, but it is not foolproof and sometimes difficulties arise in dealing with individual animals. Animals not having tuberculosis will often react to the test (false positives) while some of those with the disease may show no reaction (false negatives). There is also the problem that contact with avian type bacilli produces sensitivity to bovine tuberculin though it rarely produces widespread disease in cattle.

Extensive surveys carried out in Great Britain and Ireland have shown that 8-12 per cent of disease-free cattle give positive reactions to what is called the single tuberculin test (Lesslie and Hebert, 1975; Lesslie, Hebert and Freischs, 1976; O'Reilly and MacClancy, 1968). A comparative tuberculin test with avian and bovine tuberculins is therefore used in routine tuberculin

2. Personal communication, Dr M. Wiley, ESRI.

testing of cattle in these countries. Where this test is used two individual injections are given, one using an avian tuberculin and the other a bovine strain.

If the single intradermal test were used in Ireland on a round test where 7 million cattle are tested, between 560,000 and 840,000 disease-free cattle would be removed as reactors. This would be exceedingly wasteful. In other EEC countries the problem with non-specific infection is not so great. Only 0.5 to 1.0 per cent of tuberculosis free cattle give a positive reaction to bovine tuberculin. In these countries, therefore, the comparative test is used only as a supplementary test to determine the disease status of individual animals.

The tuberculin test is applied in a number of ways and in different sites. In general the tuberculins are injected into the thickness of the skin of the neck and the degree of resulting inflammation and swelling is established by palpation and measurement of the double thickness of the skin 72 hours after inoculation.

The reaction to the avian tuberculin acts as an index of sensitisation to antigens other than the bovine tubercle bacillus and what is regarded as the "true" reading is obtained by comparing the increase in skin thickness resulting from the avian injection with the increase in skin thickness resulting from the bovine injection. The readings from a test are interpreted from a chart which shows positive, negative and inconclusive results depending on the circumstances of the test (monitor test, reactor retest, etc.) and the interpretation adopted, whether the "standard" or the "severe" interpretation.

The EEC *standard* interpretation classifies animals as positive when the bovine reaction exceeds the avian reaction by more than 4mm, and classifies animals as inconclusive when the bovine *response* exceeds 2mm and the bovine excess (over the avian) is 1-4mm. The standard Department of Agriculture instruction advises the removal as reactors of all animals positive or inconclusive on the test when the veterinary surgeon carrying out the test is of the opinion that there is bovine infection present in a herd. In heavily infected herds further animals may be removed as reactors irrespective of the skin measurements because of clinical or epidemiological criteria. In herds where no animals are found positive to the test (as defined above) inconclusives are not removed but their cards are taken up and they are not allowed to be moved out of the herd until they are retested after an interval of 60 days. Twice inconclusive animals on the standard interpretation must be deemed positive and removed. When the inconclusives and positives on the standard EEC interpretation are removed as reactors this is referred to as applying the so-called *severe interpretation*.

For a detailed discussion of the reliability of the tuberculin test the reader is referred to Appendix A. This appendix shows that when factors other than simple skin measurements are taken into account the test can be very reliable if properly applied. Unfortunately the application is not always satisfactory. Holding facilities for animals on farms may be inadequate, the needles may be inserted at the wrong angle resulting in incomplete delivery of tuberculin at the site. In inserting the needle considerable pressure on the plunger is usually necessary. If this is not so it should be suspected that the needle has penetrated to the subcutaneous tissue, which is an incorrect procedure. Errors can easily occur also in measuring skinfold thicknesses. With careful operators these errors are minimised but with less careful people mistakes can occur. In general, unless there are proper holding facilities for the animals and unless the working area is satisfactory the operator should not carry out the test.

Vaccination of cattle with BCG (as is now a fairly general practice in humans) has been investigated widely in the past as a means of eradicating the disease but as Ritchie (1959) points out it can only be used on calves which are tuberculin negative and also if their contacts are negative. In addition it must give complete and not just partial immunity to natural infection for the rest of the vaccinate's life. Vaccinated animals become reactive to tuberculin so making further diagnostic procedures impossible. Hence Richie states that even if vaccination proved to be safe and reasonably efficient it has no place in the eradication of bovine tuberculosis and this view is generally accepted by the experts.

Methods of Eradication Using the Tuberculin Test

The incidence of tuberculosis varies under different management systems, and adjustments to the husbandry methods may help to control the disease, nevertheless "eradication will not be achieved without positive steps to eliminate infection whatever the type of herd" (Ritchie, 1959, p. 714). To this end identification of the infected animal is all important.

Eradication of bovine tuberculosis did not become a practical proposition until tuberculin was developed and adopted as a diagnostic agent. Indeed any success that has been achieved in eradicating the disease from herds or areas has depended on this method of identification of infected animals despite its drawbacks.

Where the test shows that the incidence of reactors in a herd is high (over 50 per cent) the whole herd should be slaughtered as has often been done in the later stages of an eradication campaign. When the incidence of reactors in a herd is low, however, the reactors only are removed from the herd. Disinfection of any part of buildings which may have become contaminated is carried out and manure is removed to arable land and stacked away from stock. The herd is again tested at short intervals (2 months) after disinfection has been completed so as to identify animals which were at the incubation stage and not yet tuberculin sensitive at the last testing. Routine short interval tests, removal of reactors and disinfection is repeated until infection is finally eliminated. It is also advisable to keep stock off pastures which have been grazed by reactors for several months after the latter have been removed. The bacillus causing the disease is readily killed by sunlight but can persist for long periods out of light in cattle droppings, byres and other places. Hence the need for thorough disinfection of buildings in which reactor animals are housed.

After the buildings have been swept clean of manure, straw and other loose material, the whole of the floors, walls and partitions should be scraped and scrubbed with a hot 4 per cent solution of sodium carbonate (washing soda) from a high powered sprayer. Such sprayers are now available on loan from the Irish District Veterinary Offices (DVOs). It is also important to ensure that road and rail vehicles used for the transport of tuberculosis free animals are similarly disinfected after use on each occasion.

Maintenance of Herds Free from Tuberculosis

When herds free of tuberculosis have been established it is essential to adopt strict rules for the maintenance of freedom from infection. In this context the first priority is to establish an attested herd scheme. This is a herd in which two successive tuberculin tests have revealed no reactors. If reactors are found at either of these tests a further test is carried out not less than 60 days after the removal of reactors and disinfection of premises, and the process is repeated until two tests without reactors have been made. The herd is again tested in 6 months and if this test reveals no reactors the herd is not tested again for approximately 12 months and at yearly or two-yearly intervals thereafter. Hence, when a country or area is declared free of the disease annual or biennial testing has to be carried on to maintain the position.

Indeed the fact that a country has been declared attested does not mean that bovine tuberculosis has been eradicated in a literal sense. It is doubtful in the present state of knowledge or without excessively onerous measures whether such a goal can be attained. Experience has shown that an incidence of 20 per cent of reactors in an area can easily be reduced to 0.5 per cent by repeated testing, with rapid removal of reactors, and disinfection, but any appreciable lessening of the latter figure may take a considerable time. For example, between 1941 and 1957 the animal incidence in Britain fell only from 0.41 to 0.37 (Macrae, 1961); it took a further 10 years to bring it below 0.05 per cent (Table 1).

In addition to annual rounds of testing, post-mortem examination of slaughtered animals at abbatoirs is a very important means of monitoring the extent of tuberculosis in cattle. An attested animal found on post-mortem examination to have laboratory confirmed lesions[3] should be traced back to the herd from whence it came and this herd subjected immediately to close scrutiny to determine if further animals are infected and how the infection took place. It may have resulted from a bought-in animal and if so the herd from which this animal came should be traced and so on until pockets of infection are tracked down and eliminated. It has been found in several countries, from which the disease is supposed to be eradicated, that some 0.025 per cent of attested cattle have lesions at slaughter while at round tests a similar proportion of attested animals show positive reaction. Hence careful attention must be given to the testing of herds in areas from which infection has apparently been eliminated.

Table 1: *Percentage of Cattle Reacting Positively to the Tuberculosis Test in Great Britain and South West England 1961-82*

Year	Great Britain	South West England	Year	Great Britain	South West England	Year	Great Britain	South West England
1961	0.162	0.250	1968	0.037	0.073	1975	0.038	0.098
1962	0.108	0.196	1969	0.042	0.087	1976	0.027	0.068
1963	0.068	0.096	1970	0.045	0.103	1977	0.020	0.046
1964	0.063	0.112	1971	0.038	0.110	1978	0.019	0.044
1965	0.046	0.071	1972	0.035	0.095	1979	0.018	0.036
1966	0.045	0.091	1973	0.032	0.104	1980	0.026	0.059
1967	0.049	0.097	1974	0.034	0.081	1981	0.023	0.062
						1982	0.016	0.036

Sources: Zuckerman Report and Department of Agriculture, Dublin.

If there are infected animals which show low sensitivity to tuberculin in a herd (as there generally are) then a long interval between tests will allow the infection to become active and render the animals infective. The disease will thus spread within the herd and in turn animals sold from such herds will infect herds to which they are moved. Also, it is fairly well established that inactive lesions can become active under stressful conditions such as often occur in this country where there is scarcity of winter fodder and damp lying conditions. The need for periodic testing is thus obvious and EEC Council Directive 64/432 states that *where the national incidence of infected herds is*

3. Approximately one-third of lesions discovered in slaughtered non-reactor animals are caused by pathological conditions other than tuberculosis.

over 1 per cent the official TB free status can only be maintained by an annual test. The Directive states that before a Member state can discontinue regular tuberculosis testing at least 99.9 per cent of all bovine herds should have been declared officially tuberculosis free for at least 10 years and additionally, every year for at least 6 years, bovine tuberculosis should not have been found to be present in more than 1 herd in 10,000. This may appear to be a very strict regulation, but it is inspired by the Member States who have achieved these standards themselves.

Once herds have been declared free of the disease it is most important to control the movement of animals into the herd. These must be free of infection or they will spread the disease in the attested herd. Contact between animals in attested herds and neighbouring farms has to be prevented also and in practice it has been found that a double fence may be necessary to achieve proper segregation. Substantial walls, hedges, or banks are adequate boundaries but not single wire fences or fences over which adjoining cattle can touch each other. The most important requirement, however, is that the fences are stockproof so that there is no mixing of the two classes of animals.

Other sources of re-infection include milk which has not been produced in the herd. According to Ritchie (*ibid.*, p. 725) cases are on record where milk from affected herds or even pasteurised milk purchased in bulk for calf rearing has given rise to infection in a number of animals. Another source of infection is the use by veterinary surgeons of instruments and equipment which have not been properly sterilised.

Incidence in Badgers

Other animal species such as man, badgers, deer, goats and opposums may become affected and serve as reservoirs of M. bovis in cattle. In badgers the disease usually spreads rapidly, with the lungs and kidneys (and their associated lymph nodes) being particularly vulnerable to the bovine strain of the bacillus. As a result it takes the form that can be likened to the human condition commonly known as "galloping consumption".

It is now fairly well established that badgers serve as carriers of the bovine tubercle bacillus and are likely to infect cattle in areas where there are high badger and cattle densities as, for example, in South West England and probably in many parts of Ireland.

The Badger Situation in Britain

Following complete attestation in Great Britain in 1960 the reactor incidence persisted at a higher level in certain areas in South West England than in the rest of the country. Because of this persistence a departmental team conducted an inquiry in order to establish reasons for the high infection rate among cattle. Their findings were reported to the Chief Veterinary Officer of the Ministry of Agriculture, Fisheries and Food (MAFF) in 1972 but their recommendations proved to be of little practical value. The most important recommendation was to increase the frequency of testing in order to detect the disease before it had time to spread. The application of this recommendation, however, failed to resolve the problem (Evans and Thompson, 1980).

In April 1971 while the departmental inquiry was being conducted a dead badger was found on a farm in Gloucestershire where infected cattle had been disclosed at a recent test. Typical lesions of tuberculosis were found in the lungs and other organs of this badger and M. bovis was isolated from them. By December 1972 four other infected badgers were found in the same area and a survey around that time found that the infection rate in badgers was 28.3 per cent in the Dursley/Wotton area of Gloucestershire.

In experiments carried out at the Central Veterinary Laboratory, Weybridge, in 1976, it was demonstrated that badgers became infected after inoculation with doses of M. bovis isolated from cattle and that healthy badgers in contact with inoculated badgers became infected. Calves kept in contact with these badgers reacted to the tuberculin test and on post-mortem examination lesions of tuberculosis were found and M. bovis isolated. However, the reaction in calves only occurred after, at least, 6 months' contact. These experiments indicated the likelihood that transmission of M. bovis can occur from badger to badger and from badger to cattle. A Committee under the Chairmanship of Lord Zuckerman which reported in 1980 (Zuckerman, 1980) concluded that badgers were and are responsible for the relatively high incidence of the disease in South West England where there are heavy densities of both cattle and badgers. Attempts, however, to eliminate badgers in this region were strongly resisted by the wild animal preservation societies and the relatively high incidence of the disease continues to persist in the area. Whether it would decline if badgers were eliminated entirely is not universally agreed. Wilesmith (1983) says that "in this field the relative risk of cattle acquiring infection from badgers is low and usually only a small number of cattle become infected". The annual incidence of the disease in Britain and in the southwest of England for the years 1961-1982 is shown in Table 1.

The Dunnet Report

One of the recommendations in Lord Zuckerman's report was that there should be a further overall review 3 years after his own findings were published. In September 1984 the Minister for Agriculture, Fisheries and Food, the Rt. Hon. Michael Jopling, announced that he and the Secretary of State for Wales, the Rt. Hon. Nicholas Edwards, had set up another Committee to review the situation. This Committee consisted of Professor G.M. Dunnet, Regius Professor of Natural History at the University of Aberdeen, Chairman, Mr D.M. Jones, Director of Zoos of the Zoological Society of London and Professor J.P. McInerney, Glenely Professor of Agricultural Policy at the University of Exeter. This Committee which has now issued its report (Dunnet, *et al.*, March, 1986) is much less definite than Lord Zuckerman's about the role of badgers in herd break-down. It makes the following recommendations, among others:

(1) Though badgers may constitute the main source of re-infection of cattle with bovine tuberculosis we cannot over-emphasise that there are still many gaps in our knowledge of the epidemiology of the disease in badgers.

(2) For the time being action should be taken against badgers, only after a herd break-down for which no other source of infection can be found, in areas of the country where there has been a recent history of herd break-down which has been attributed to infected badgers.

(3) In such circumstances the badgers using that part of the farm where it is believed that the disease was transmitted to cattle, or the whole farm if it is not possible to be more precise, should be captured, killed humanely and examined post mortem, without prior sampling or delineation of social groups and with no question of extending the operation beyond the breakdown farm. The policy of clearing whole areas of badgers by gassing or otherwise is to be discontinued.

(4) The Ministry should keep the badger control strategy under continuous review and in particular reconsider it if (a) no infection is found in the badgers removed in a significant number of cases or (b) there is evidence of a significant increase in herd break-downs.

(5) The Ministry encourages farmers to seek to prevent (a) cattle having access to badger setts (through the erection of wire fencing) or (b) as far as possible prevent badgers and cattle eating from the same food source (i.e., grain troughs in fields).

In view of these recommendations it is obvious that the role of the badger in the transmission of bovine tuberculosis is far from settled and wholesale removal of badgers is no longer being recommended.

Incidence in Other Animals
Infected cattle are a source of infection for pigs and the incidence of

bovine tuberculosis in pigs has been reduced *pari passu* with the progress of tuberculosis eradication in cattle. Domestic poultry and other birds are also troublesome in that they will infect cattle, particularly calves, with the avian type of organism which may set up small localised lesions in the bovine. These are not considered to be harmful and for that reason the comparative test (described above) which is of assistance in differentiating between the bovine and avian type of infection has been developed.

Contact with infected animals and the drinking of unpasteurised milk from tuberculosis cows can give rise to the disease in humans and many people are fearful of contacting the disease in this way. Infected farm workers may also infect cattle. If a worker is infected with the bovine type of organism it will establish itself in the cattle he tends and will spread rapidly through the herd. Furthermore, exposure of cattle to human type tubercle bacilli may succeed in making animals sensitive to the bovine tuberculin test in such a way that it is extremely difficult to differentiate from true bovine tuberculosis. Only rarely, however, has infection caused by the human type of organism been demonstrated in cattle in Ireland or Great Britain although in northern Europe the condition was reported frequently in the 1930s. However, repeated tests in most countries have shown that the most serious risk of re-infection in cattle is directly or indirectly from other infected cattle and obviously the establishment of more and more tuberculosis free herds in a locality reduces the risk. Unfortunately, in many European countries while it was optional for farmers to eliminate the disease a large number of infected herds remained. It was for that reason that eradication had to be made compulsory and compensation paid to farmers for losses incurred on the disposal of reactor cattle.

Incentives to Eradication

The pressure to eradicate bovine tuberculosis has arisen for a variety of reasons. In most countries where the incidence was high, the public health aspect had a marked influence and the early endeavour had been to supply safe milk, especially for children. The amount of beef condemned in abbatoirs because of tuberculosis has also affected the position. Most important, however, has been the serious loss to agriculture from clinical and subclinical tuberculosis in cattle (wasting) and certainly this has had a more direct effect on farming opinion. In Ireland, especially, there have also been strong external market pressures. Most of our EEC partners and the USA have now eliminated bovine tuberculosis (see Table 2).

The Epidemiology of Tuberculosis Contrasted with that of Brucellosis

The brucellosis eradication scheme which commenced in Ireland in 1965 was completed in 1986 with the disease eradicated, for all practical purposes.

Table 2: *Position Regarding Bovine Tuberculosis in EC Member States and in USA in 1985*

Member State	Position in Regard to BTE	Member State	Position in Regard to BTE
Denmark	Eradicated	UK*	Practically eradicated
Holland	Eradicated (30 cases a year)	Italy	77 per cent of herds are classed officially free, 27,884 reactors in 1984
Luxembourg	Eradicated	Ireland	97.6 per cent of herds are classed officially free, 31,572 reactors in 1985
W. Germany	Eradicated (about 20 cases a year)		
France	99 per cent of herds are classed officially free, 17,330 reactors in 1984		
		Greece	82 per cent of herds are classed officially free
Spain	67 per cent of herds are classed officially free, 73,698 reactors in 1985	Portugal	75 per cent of herds are classed officially free
Belgium	Practically eradicated	USA**	Practically eliminated

* In Northern Ireland the herd incidence was 1.6 per cent in 1984. There is, however, difficulty in keeping the disease at this level because *inter alia* (it is claimed) of imports from the Republic.

** At the time official control began in the USA in 1917 the prevalence of the disease in cattle was about 5 per cent. By 1969 this had been reduced to 0.08 per cent. In 1917 one beef carcase, out of every 188 examined at slaughter, was found to have generalised tuberculosis. By 1969, 390,000 cattle carcases were examined for every generalised case found. In the early years of the programme detection was mainly by mass tuberculin testing of the cattle population. In 1960 detection relied increasingly on traceback of deceased animals from slaughterhouses to their premises of origin (Shwabe, 1984).

Source: Department of Agriculture.

The ordinary layperson often wonders why bovine tuberculosis could not have been cleared up in the same length of time. The main differences between the two diseases are contrasted in Appendix C.

It is obvious from the discussion in Appendix C that bovine tuberculosis is a very difficult disease to clear up as, indeed, is human tuberculosis. In Britain it took 27 years to get the incidence down to acceptable levels (less than 0.05 per cent of animals). The time taken in the USA was about 50 years but like Ireland there were difficulties in that country with cattle movement in the ranching states and with cross border movement from Mexico. In Northern Ireland it took 22 years to get the animal incidence down to 0.04 per cent, but when in 1971 triennial testing was introduced the incidence rose again and annual testing had to be resumed in 1982 (see Chapter 2 and Table 8). In Israel eradication started in 1952 and by 1965 the animal incidence was down to 0.01 per cent. Attention was relaxed at that stage and there was a gradual rise to 0.11 per cent in 1968 and it has not been reduced below that level since then. Testing commenced in New Zealand in 1958 and the disease is still not eradicated in that country. In Ireland the animal incidence appears to be at about 0.2 per cent which is more than four times what we would wish it to be, despite over 30 years' testing and removal of reactors.

Chapter 2

HISTORY OF THE BOVINE TUBERCULOSIS ERADICATION SCHEME IN IRELAND

In the years prior to 1954, bovine tuberculosis was by far the most serious livestock disease in Ireland. The disease, apart from its implications for human health, was severely limiting the productivity of the country's cattle stocks. By that time also the eradication of the disease had become necessary to safeguard Ireland's store cattle export trade with Great Britain (Watchorn, 1965). This trade was a dominant item in the economy. In 1954 the value of Irish store cattle exports represented over 20 per cent of the total value of Irish exports to all countries (£111.5m out of £485m).

An eradication scheme had been started in Britain in 1935, and despite the war years, about 50 per cent of the herds in that country had been attested (certified clear of the disease) by 1954. Furthermore, the plan for area attestation was under way in Scotland, Wales and Northern England where some counties had already become attested areas. The day was therefore coming when all Irish store cattle exported to Britain would have to be of attested status.

The problems of the eradication of bovine tubulercosis on a national scale in Ireland had been under investigation for a considerable period. A pilot study of eradication had been in progress in Bansha in South Tipperary since 1950. This scheme had proved most useful and informative in indicating the general pattern on which eradication methods in this country should be based. In line with the developments in other countries, it showed that the campaign should be on the basis of clearing whole areas at a time.

It was realised from the start that the scheme would take many years to bring to completion. All 250,000 cattle herds in the State would have to be brought under a continuing system of testing, reactors would have to be removed, sales of cattle at farms and markets regulated and inter-herd movements of cattle controlled. No other scheme previously undertaken by the Department was of such magnitude.

The eradication programme in Ireland can be divided into two periods. The first period runs from 1954 when the scheme was initiated, up to 1965 when the whole State was declared officially free of the disease by the Minister

25

for Agriculture. The second period runs from 1965 to the present time when there is still a relatively high incidence of the disease in the State.

Period 1954-1965

The eradication scheme during this period has been described in detail by Watchorn (1965) and the main features only are summarised here.

The scheme operated in Ireland differed fundamentally from that in operation in Britain. The British scheme was based on the attestation of individual herds by the voluntary efforts of the herdowners. When at least 80 per cent of all herds in an area had become attested in this way, compulsion was applied to the remaining herds in the area and when they were cleared (on the basis of three consecutive clear tests for each herd) the area was declared an attested area. The herdowner in Britain had to have all the necessary tuberculin testing carried out and all reactors got rid of at his own expense until his herd had two consecutive clear tests. When this stage was reached, the Ministry came into the picture for the first time and if the herd then passed an official test, it became what was called "attested". The herdowner was then rewarded by bonus payments based upon either the number of cattle in the herd or the gallonage of milk sold. The bonus was at the rate of £2 per head of cattle each year (or 2p per gallon of milk) for 4 years, followed by £1 per head of cattle each year (or 1p per gallon of milk) for a further 2 years.

Eradication in Ireland was based on the clearance of an area (consisting of a county or group of counties) at a time. The disease incidence in the selected area was gradually reduced until the point was reached when the area could be declared attested. The requisite services to enable herds to be cleared of the disease were provided free of charge to the herdowners from the outset. The main facilities provided were free tuberculin testing by the veterinary surgeon (VS) of the herdowners' choice and the purchase of reactors by the Department at full current market value. There were also special grants for the erection of byres and the installation of water on farms, and grants for the installation of pasteurising equipment at creamery premises so that skim milk returned to farms would be TB free. Also, a Guaranteed Payments Scheme which operated from July 1960 to March 1962 was introduced to facilitate the marketing of cattle which could not be exported as stores because of attestation in Britain. As most of Britain became attested, Irish stores were not allowed on to farms and so cattle had to be exported as fat animals for direct slaughter or as dead meat. In both these cases, prices were lower than the corresponding prices for stores which were linked to the British fatstock Deficiency Payments Scheme.

There were four stages under the Irish scheme, viz., (a) Voluntary, (b) Clearance, (c) Blue Card, and (d) Attestation.

Voluntary stage: Under the voluntary stage it was open to any herdowner in a selected area to participate in the eradication measures, the facilities provided being free testing and compensation at full market value for reactors purchased by the Department.

Clearance stage: When the disease incidence in an area was reduced sufficiently by voluntary effort, the area was declared a clearance area and thenceforward the eradication measures were on a compulsory basis. All herds had to be tested, all reactors removed and the movement of cattle into the area and between herds was strictly controlled. All cattle were given a special ear-tag for the purpose of identification when the first compulsory herd test was carried out. Each tag had a code number for the county in which it was first affixed together with a serial number.

Animal identification card (blue card) stage: Herds in clearance areas which had passed the second of three clearance tests qualified for the issue of animal identification cards (blue cards) which conferred a certain status on the cattle in these herds (i.e., 14-day tested). These cattle could be exported under permit without further testing.

The blue card is and was equivalent to a passport for each individual animal. When issued, it showed the herd number, ear-tag number, colour, breed, sex and date of the last test of the herd in which the animal was tested. At the commencement of each subsequent test of the herd the veterinary surgeon took up the cards. If all the animals passed the test he entered the date of the test, the herd number and his signature on each card. He then handed the cards back to the herdowner. If all the animals did not pass the test, the VS sent all the cards with his report to the District Office and the cards were not restored to the herdowner until further testing had shown that the herd was clear again. This procedure is still in operation. Nowadays the herd is said to be "locked up" during the period when the identification cards are in the District Office and animals in that herd may not be moved to fairs or marts or allowed to mix with other herds. Contiguous herds are also tested at this time to locate any lateral spread from the originally restricted herd.

Each identification card has its own serial number and each district veterinary office maintains a register of the cards issued in that district. This system, along with the ear-tag number, enables every animal to be traced back to every herd in which it was tested. Hence, if a slaughtered animal is found to have TB lesions, it can be traced back through the District Office to the herds in which it was tested so that these herds can be investigated. In recent years, however, it has become apparent that the blue card method of trace-back is very deficient. Through it animals can be traced back only to the herds in which they were tested; herds in which they were located but not tested cannot be identified.

Attested stage: During the clearance and blue card stages in an area, the controls on the movement and sale of cattle were made progressively stiffer and restrictions were imposed on herds in areas where the incidence of tuberculosis had not been sufficiently reduced. Area attestation was granted when the third round of clearance testing had been completed if it had shown that TB had become virtually non-existent in the area. Within an attested area animals could move freely between herds and to and from sales. In order to protect the status of herds in the area, however, the movement of cattle into the area had to be controlled. Cattle leaving the area could do so only under permit and had to move under conditions of strict isolation so that they could retain their attested status.

Progress of the Scheme

The scheme started in September 1954 with intensive measures on a voluntary scale in Clare and Sligo and the Bansha area in Tipperary, the main incentives offered in these areas being free testing and the purchase of reactors by the Department. At the same time herdowners in the other 24 counties were offered free testing. The byre, water and pasteurisation grants mentioned above were made generally available at this time also.

Testing carried out during the first year indicated that the overall herd incidence of the disease was 17 per cent and that it was much higher in cows (22%) than in other cattle (8%). It also became evident that the disease was much less prevalent in the western and midland areas than in the southern dairying counties. The overall herd incidence was found to be 6 per cent in the west, 12 per cent in the midlands and 26 per cent in the south.[4]

Over the years, the compulsory scheme was gradually introduced first in the west, midlands and east of the country and finally in the 6 dairying counties of Cork, Kerry, Kilkenny, Limerick, Tipperary and Waterford. From the inception of the eradication programme it had always been realised that the high incidence of disease in the latter counties and the dependence of the area on dairying would present the most complex problems. A special southern scheme introduced in these counties in 1959 and terminated in 1962 effected a reduction in the overall incidence of the disease from 34 per cent in cows in 1954 to 11 per cent by mid-1962. In this effort 265,000 cow reactors were removed and over 32,000 herds were declared clear. The final drive was

4. These are likely to be minimum figures in the context of current testing and other detection procedures.

commenced in this area in 1962 and after four rounds of testing the southern dairying counties were declared attested on 19 October 1965. This completed the attestation of the entire country just 11 years after the start of the eradication campaign in 1954. Unfortunately the disease was not by any means cleared up at that time as subsequent events showed.

Period 1966 to Date

When the country was declared an attested area (virtually disease free) in 1965 the incidence of tuberculosis in herds was just over 2 per cent compared with 17 per cent 12 years previously. This amounted to considerable progress since the scheme was initiated. Unfortunately, the impetus was not sustained in later years: the incidence on the 1982 round of testing was virtually identical with that disclosed in the 1966 round (see Table 3) and was much higher than this in most of the intervening years. Nor has there been any sustained improvement since 1982. The incidence increased to 3.2 per cent in 1983, improved to 2.24 per cent in 1984 but increased again to 3.2 per cent at the end of 1985.

The figures for incidence or indeed for any other measure must, however, be interpreted with caution. As explained in a later section of this chapter, they are not comparable from year to year because of different testing intensities in the different years.

Table 3: *TB Incidence Levels on Annual Round Testing and Number of Reactors Removed 1966-1985*

Year	Incidence of Disease (%)		No. of Reactors Removed	Year	Incidence of Disease (%)		No. of Reactors Removed
	In Herds	In Animals			In Herds	In Animals	
1966	2.80	0.28	23,378	1976	n.a.	n.a.	24,888
1967	3.29	0.34	25,862	1977	7.5	0.55	51,268
1968	3.30	0.31	22,021	1978	n.a.	n.a.	31,238
1969	4.40	0.42	31,060	1979	3.95	0.25	21,483
1970	4.49	0.40	37,104	1980	2.94	0.19	26,581
1971	4.12	0.37	37,408	1981	2.11	0.16	29,755
1972	4.50	0.37	31,258	1982	2.76	0.20	26,700
1973	4.84	0.35	36,687	1983	3.16	n.c.	27,691
1974	5.11	0.42	46,656	1984	2.24	n.c.	33,560
1975	n.a.	n.a.	21,339	1985	3.19	n.c.	34,404

n.a.: Not available due to veterinary dispute.   n.c.: not computed.
Source: Department of Agriculture.

Cost to Exchequer 1954-65

The data in Table 4 indicate the scale of the operation from the time the scheme started in 1954 until the whole State was declared an attested area in 1965. Net expenditure on the scheme during this period (gross less salvage realisation on reactors of £16.9 million) was £37.9 million. Of this, £19.4 million was paid to herdowners in respect of reactors, £11.0 million went in veterinary surgeons' fees. One million was spent on grants for byres, water installation on farms and pasteurisation equipment in creameries, while the remaining £6.5 million went on other expenses. These included travelling expenses, publicity and supplies of tuberculin, ear-tags and stationery, etc., but not the salaries of Departmental staff employed on the scheme. The largest item under other expenses was £4.5 million spent on guarantee payments to facilitate the marketing of cattle which could not be exported as stores because of attestation in Britain. The total net cost at 1985 prices (based on the Consumer Price Index) was £368.8 million.

Table 4: *Government Expenditure Each Year on BTE Scheme 1954/55 to 1965/66 at Current and Constant 1985 Prices*

Year	Payment for Reactors Net	VS Fees	Byre Grants & Water	Other Items	Total Current	Total at 1985 Prices**
			£'000			
1954/55	37.5	48.9	—	11.6	98.0	1,159.1
1955/56	24.9	121.6	31.5	34.6	212.6	2,475.4
1956/57	61.2	210.0	169.4	36.8	477.4	5,295.7
1957/58	146.7	264.2	149.5	38.7	599.1	6,278.7
1958/59	487.5	476.1	117.0	88.0	1,168.6	11,953.9
1959/60	3,783.2	1,045.0	105.9	149.9	5,084.0	52,590.4
1960/61	2,991.0	1,272.9	136.6	526.0*	4,926.5	50,265.4
1961/62	2,826.8	1,477.4	122.7	4,509.9*	8,936.8	88,685.7
1962/63	4,385.2	1,624.1	151.4	431.8*	6,592.5	62,615.7
1963/64	2,763.3	1,459.9	n.a.	429.5	4,652.7	43,705.4
1964/65	1,354.5	1,615.9	n.a.	148.5	3,118.9	26,870.2
1965/66	538.8	1,368.2	n.a.	140.8	2,047.8	16,911.3
Total	19,400.6	10,984.2	984.0	6,546.1	37,914.9	368,806.9
Per cent	51.2	29.0	2.6	17.3	100	—

*Includes guarantee payments to facilitate the marketing of cattle which could not be exported as stores because of attestation in Britain.
**Current prices adjusted by Consumer Price Index.
Source: Department of Agriculture.

During the period of the campaign, some 600 private veterinary surgeons were engaged almost continuously on testing. The Department's technical staff (not all of whom were engaged wholetime on the BTE scheme) consisted of 24 veterinary officers, 18 supervisory officers and 305 lay staff, while on the administrative side, 210 officers were employed, over 160 of whom were located in 17 District Offices throughout the country. The total number of reactors removed from herds in the course of the campaign was 831,000. Of these, 567,000 were purchased directly by the Department and disposed of by contract to licensed canneries and meat factories.

Costs 1954-85

The costs from 1966/67 to date are given in Table 5. This table shows that in the period 1966 to 1985 a total of £149.7 million was spent on efforts to eradicate bovine tuberculosis. When this is added to the total current expenditure from Table 4, the overall figure comes to £187.6 million which is equivalent to £730 million at 1985 prices. This is somewhat of an over-statement of the cost to the Irish taxpayer however. In 1984 and 1985 disease levies paid by farmers were £5.9 and £13.0 million respectively, while a further £9.5 million was obtained from the EEC in the period 1978 to 1981 (see Chapter 3). Hence the net exchequer cost over the whole period at 1985 prices was about £692 million.

Of the total expenditure given in Table 5, 40.6 per cent went on payments for reactors, 43.7 per cent was spent on veterinary fees and the remaining 15.7 per cent on tuberculin, ear-tags, publicity and the travelling expenses of Department officers in connection with the scheme.

Figures are not given on a regular basis for the number of veterinary surgeons employed on testing but, taking the most recent figure available of 860 and dividing it into the veterinary fees for 1985, we obtain an average fee per veterinary surgeon of about £13,000 in that year. The figure for 1984 estimated at 1985 prices was about £9,000.

The figures for the costs of the disease in Table 5 are minimum figures since they do not include the salaries of the Departmental staff employed on the scheme (about 1,300) either in Dublin or in the District Offices. As these people were also employed on the brucellosis scheme over the past 20 years or so, it is difficult to allocate their salaries. The total administration costs of these two schemes since their inception was £108 million. When this is raised to 1985 prices it comes to £256 million and when divided in proportion to direct expenditure on the two schemes the administration of the tuberculosis scheme from 1954 to 1985 comes to £173 million at 1985 prices. This would bring the total cost (less farmers' levies and EEC payments) over the period to about £865 million or an average cost per annum of around £27 million.

Table 5: *Government Expenditure Each Year on the BTE Scheme 1966-67 to 1985**

Year	Payment for Reactors (Net)	VS Fees	Other Payments	Total Payments	
				At Current Prices	At 1985 Prices
			£'000		
1966-67	501.5	1,344.5	100.5	1,946.5	15,517.5
1967-68	719.7	1,278.5	105.2	2,103.4	16,407.3
1968-69	670.3	1,572.8	115.7	2,358.8	17,596.1
1969-70	877.0	1,420.7	196.5	2,494.2	17,160.9
1970-71	1,206.5	1,554.1	188.6	2,949.2	18,719.0
1971-72	1,569.1	1,630.9	259.5	3,459.5	20.179.9
1972-73	2,245.3	2,110.1	293.3	4,648.7	24,905.5
1973-74	3,204.2	2,036.6	259.0	5,499.8	26,486.7
1974	3,031.9	1,561.7	268.5	4,862.1	20,258.2
1975	2,456.1	787.8	419.2	3,663.1	12,627.1
1976	1,192.1	465.1	419.7	2,076.9	6,067.8
1977	3,902.9	2,976.7	771.2	7,650.8	19,666.4
1978	3,422.9	3,347.8	998.3	7,769.0	18,558.1
1979	2,825.7	2,672.3	1,291.9	6,789.9	14,322.4
1980	2,862.1	6,520.0	1,585.6	10,967.7	19,569.0
1981	3,570.0	6,991.0	2,130.0	12,691.0	18,805.3
1982	3,684.0	7,558.0	2,240.0	13,482.0	17,056.5
1983	4,688.0	7,619.0	2,763.0	15,070.0	17,257.9
1984	6,707.0*	7,112.0	3,129.0	16,948.0	17,873.2
1985	7,419.2*	10,423.0	4,439.7	22,281.9	22,281.9
Total above	56,755.5	70,982.6	21,974.4	149.712.5	361,316.7
1954-1966	19,400.6	10,984.2	7,530.1	37,914.9	368,806.9
1954-1985	76,156.1	81,966.8	29,504.5	187,627.4	730,123.6

*Levies paid by farmers towards the cost of the scheme were £5.9 million in 1984 and £13.0 million in 1985. These amounts are not deducted in this table, nor are payments of £9.5 million received from the EEC in respect of the period 1978-1981.
Source: Department of Agriculture.

In addition to the known cost to the exchequer, there has also been the loss to the economy from the scheme. Each year has seen the slaughter of large numbers of reactors, 50 per cent of which are cows and heifers in calf. This puts a serious drain on the expansion of the national cattle herd. There is a loss of options due to the disease for greater improvement of the national herd through voluntary culling and there is also a loss due to the disruption of farm plans.

The Measurement of Tuberculosis Infection

Two measures of the level of TB infection are used, namely, *Incidence* and *Prevalence*. *Incidence* is the number of herds or animals in the State which break down in any year as a proportion of the number of non-restricted herds or animals in the State tested in that year. *Prevalence* is the number of herds found to be infected during the year as a percentage of the total number of herds in the State. This is period prevalence. Point prevalence is the total number of herds restricted at any one point in time as a percentage of the total number of herds in the State.

Both these measures are deficient, particularly in a year when all the herds in the State are not tested. The prevalence measure is particularly defective in such a year because it relates the number of restricted herds to the total number of herds in the State. If, say, only half the herds are tested in a year, as has happened in some years, then the number of infected herds must be understated and the prevalence lower than it would be if all herds were tested. Hence the prevalence figure is accurate only if all the herds are tested and even then the figures may not be comparable from year to year. In a period when there is a full round of testing as well as intensive testing of heavily infected areas a relatively large number of reactors will be picked up and the number of herds restricted in that period will be higher than in years when funds are scarcer and testing of infected areas is not so intensive.

The incidence figures can also be unreliable, both in years when full rounds of testing take place as well as in other years. The following figures for 1983 when a full round of testing took place explain how difficult it is to get accurate results using either of the measures.

Number of reactor herds	9,856
Revealed as follows:	
Round tests	3,883
Six-month check test	315
Special check test	1,764
Inconclusive second tests	2,178
Private (pre-movement) tests	739
Factory reactors	977
Total number of herds in State	195,488
Herds tested on round	164,153

Actual incidence quoted for round = 3,883/164,153 = 2.23%

It is obvious that the incidence figure is very low because it related to all the fairly good herds, i.e., 3,883 reactor herds were revealed in 164,153 herds tested on the round, whereas there were 5,973 reactor herds among the remaining 31,335 herds which were tested outside the round. The incidence in these herds (though officially it is not classed as incidence) was 5,973/ 31,335 = 19.1 per cent. Certainly the prevalence figure is the most reliable in this year since it relates the total number of infected herds found during the year to the total number of herds. It is 9,856/195,488 = 5.04 per cent, much higher than the incidence figure, though probably too high because there was intensive testing in that year. Hence, in a year when there is a full round of testing as well as intensive testing of black spots, the prevalence figure is too high and the incidence figure too low. On the other hand, in a year when there is not a full round of testing the bad areas only will be tested, both in round and check tests, and in that year the incidence figure will be much higher than in a year when there is a full round, while the prevalence figure will be lower. The comparability of the figures, therefore, from year to year is suspect, regardless of whether we use prevalence or incidence. How then do we get over this problem? For statistical purposes there is only one way of doing this; a random sample of herds must be tested on a uniform basis every year regardless of whether full or partial rounds of testing are being undertaken.

To obtain fairly accurate figures (+ or - 1%) on a county basis at the present time (when the "incidence" of the disease is around 2 per cent) the sample size would need to be about 15,000 herds, with roughly about 500 herds sampled in each county or part of a county. Some of the herds in the sample would probably coincide with herds due for testing as part of the programme, but these herds should, for uniformity, be tested by a Departmental veterinarian. As the incidence of the disease is reduced over time, the size of the sample would have to be increased. If the incidence were halved from 2 per cent to 1 per cent, the sample size would have to be doubled. Hence, when the incidence gets very low, sample testing to determine incidence on a country basis would not be justified. The sample size would have to be too large. If, however, we are interested only in the overall national incidence, a much smaller sample (2,000 herds or so) would suffice at the present time, but by the time the national herd incidence were reduced to 0.5 per cent, the sample size would have to be very large. At that stage full rounds of testing every few years would have to be carried out to monitor incidence.

Herd and Animal Incidence

The publication of official figures for herd rather than for animal incidence tends to be somewhat misleading as it takes no account of herd size. Animal incidence or prevalence is a more accurate representation of the situation and even though EEC definitions relate to herds the Department should change over to publication of both animal and herd figures.

Incidence of Lesions in Non-Reactor Cattle

In the absence of random sampling of herds for testing, the incidence of lesions in non-reactor cattle slaughtered is usually taken to be the most reliable figure for judging the incidence of the disease in the State.

Figures for such incidence are given in Table 6 where they are compared with animal incidence from testing. This table shows that the percentage of cattle showing up with lesions at meat factories has remained fairly constant at about 0.20 per cent since 1971 with a substantial rise to 0.41 per cent in 1976 coinciding with the veterinary strike at that time. The animal incidence from testing, on the other hand, would appear to have fallen over the same period but we cannot be too sure of this for the reasons given later. One point is clear from both sets of figures. The incidence rises during a period when testing is suspended. The lesion data show a rise to 0.41 per cent in 1976 at a time when testing was suspended for nearly 2 years; the incidence figures show a corresponding rise in 1977 when testing was resumed after the strike.

Table 6: *Lesions in Non-Reactor Cattle at Registered Meat Factories Compared with Incidence from Testing 1971-1984*

Year	Percentage with Lesions	Animal Incidence from Testing	Year	Percentage with Lesions	Animal Incidence from Testing
1971	0.20	0.37	1978	0.28	n.a.
1972	0.21	0.37	1979	0.23	0.25
1973	0.24	0.35	1980	0.20	0.19
1974	0.20	0.42	1981	0.25	0.16
1975	0.23	n.a.	1982	0.20	0.20
1976	0.41	n.a.	1983	0.19	n.a.
1977	0.32	0.55	1984	0.21	n.a.

Source: Department of Agriculture.

Incidence of Lesions in Reactor Cattle

Another set of figures which gives some clue to the situation is the number of reactor cattle found with tuberculosis lesions on slaughter. These figures, which are given in Table 7, show that the proportion of slaughtered reactor cattle with lesions was only about 16 per cent in 1974, but had risen erratically over the years to 36 per cent in 1984. On the basis of these data it would seem, to the layperson at any rate, that large numbers of uninfected cattle are being removed each year and that the test is over-specific. The experts, however, would not agree with this thesis. The veterinarians to whom I have spoken say that if a high proportion of reactors have no visible lesions (NVL) this does not mean that these animals are not infected. Lesions can easily be missed as cattle and organs pass through the line, sometimes at the rate of 60-80 per hour. In many of the NVL reactors passing through the line, lesions can be found at proper post mortems, and in others, small naked eye lesions can be found in the lymph nodes when sliced open with a scalpel, while others are infected but are in the pre-lesion stage (particularly if there is annual round testing). The test, for all its alleged faults, can be very sensitive and will pick up the disease at a very early stage (long before lesions occur). Some non-infected animals are, however, always removed as reactors since in heavily infected herds, animals in contact with reactors are removed also and some of these may not have the disease; some animals have great resistance to tuberculosis if they are well fed and are not under stress.

Table 7: *TB Lesions in Reactor Cattle*

Year	No. of Reactors	No. with Lesions	% with Lesions	Year	No. of Reactors	No. with Lesions	% with Lesions
1971	36,644	6,002	16.38	1979	23,637	6,950	29.40
1972	30,133	7,016	23.28	1980	29,482	6,981	23.68
1973	38,849	8,872	23.84	1981	31,857	7,300	22.91
1974	47,714	7,590	15.91	1982	31,530	7,478	23.72
1975	23,890	4,481	18.76	1983	32,294	9,170	28.40
1976	23,135	5,428	23.46	1984	33,743	12,205	36.17
1977	49,759	12,062	24.24	1985	34,498	11,103	32.18
1978	32,295	9,261	28.68				

Source: Department of Agriculture.

O'Reilly (1969a, p. 39) says that as the incidence of tuberculosis falls in a cattle population, there is a marked increase in the percentage of NVL reactors. For example, in the USA in 1959 when the incidence of the disease in herds was 0.23 per cent, 57.6 per cent of reactors were classed as NVLs. In 1963 the corresponding figures were 0.10 per cent and 75 per cent, respectively. At the present time when the incidence of the disease is very low, over 80 per cent of reactors in the US are NVL. The fact that the proportion of Irish reactors with visible lesions is tending to increase is therefore not a good sign. It means that incidence of the disease in the cattle population is, if anything, tending to increase also. However, despite what the experts say, one would have an uneasy feeling that we are removing far more non-infected cattle than we should be and that the matter should be looked at carefully by the veterinary research people to see if there is any pattern about these removals. If a high proportion is coming from the relatively clear areas of the country it could mean that the standards of interpretation are too severe in these places and would need to be relaxed.

The BTE Scheme in Northern Ireland

A summary of the BTE scheme in Northern Ireland is given below in order to show how our neighbours have progressed in this regard.

First steps to eradicate the disease were, as in Britain, taken through a voluntary attested herds scheme in 1949. At that time it is estimated that 25 per cent of animals were affected. The Scheme began slowly but over the years it gathered momentum as the effects of bonus payments began to filter back to farmers. Finally, in 1960, Northern Ireland was declared an attested area. After this date the national herd was largely on annual testing, and, with a continual decline in disease incidence, the testing interval was increased to 2 years in 1965 (biennial testing). The favourable trend in the disease level continued and in 1971 triennial testing was introduced but the herds owned by cattle dealers were always kept on annual testing.

The experts (Sullivan, 1979) say that with the benefit of hindsight, it is now clear that moving from biennial to triennial testing was premature. The downward trend in the disease level in the national herd levelled out and then started to climb (see Table 8). The decision to move to triennial testing was taken in the knowledge that the level of bovine tuberculosis was very low and also on the information that the level was decreasing in the Republic from where the vast majority of Northern cattle imports come. With triennial testing, any disease that was present had a much longer time to incubate and in 1975 it was deemed necessary to take precautionary steps immediately and to revert to biennial testing. At that time, 2.76 per cent of herds were estimated to be infected.

As well as the re-introduction of biennial testing to reduce the level of the disease, the Northern Ireland Department of Agriculture decided to raise the health standards which animals must achieve before they could be imported from the Republic. All such cattle, in addition to being of attested status, must now pass the single tuberculin test[5] within 30 days prior to being imported. Where possible, heifers are followed up and check-tested not earlier than 2 months after importation. Where staff are available, steers are also check-tested.

The national herd is back under annual testing since 1982 but several herds are currently tested more frequently than that. Dealers' herds are tested

5. This is the EEC test described in Chapter 3.

Table 8: *Progress in the Eradication of Bovine Tuberculosis in Northern Ireland 1961-1984*

Year	Cattle Tested ('000)	Reactors (No.)	Cattle Incidence[a] %	Herd Incidence[a] %	Net Expenditure[b] £'000	Comments
1961	1,000	390	0.39	—	1,468	Annual testing
1962	1,000	1,822	0.18	—	1,303	until 31-12-64
1963	1,000	1,040	0.10	—	1,194	
1964	1,000	732	0.07	—	1,020	
1965	600	487	0.08	—	461	Biennial testing
1966	600	530	0.09	—	141	from 1-1-65
1967	600	739	0.12	—	123	
1968	500	319	0.06	—	115	
1969	600	351	0.059	0.808	115	
1970	600	241	0.040	0.497	121	
1971	462	174	0.038	0.544	69	Triennial testing
1972	504	343	0.068	0.808	78	from 1-1-71
1973	614	677	0.110	1.110	111	
1974	648	834	0.129	1.509	99	
1975	709	1,178	0.166	2.756	177	
1976	772	1,475	0.191	2.435	490	Biennial testing
1977	873	1,473	0.169	2.571	686	from 1-4-76
1978	925	1,291	0.140	1.892	644	
1979	932	1,150	0.123	1.654	928	
1980	1,022	1,790	0.175	2.407	1,329	
1981	1,139	1,642	0.144	2.035	1,465	
1982	1,293	1,499	0.116	1.885	1,928	Annual testing
1983	1,688	1,802	0.107	1.775	2,404	from 8-82
1984	1,682	1,494	0.089	1.610	2,556	

(a)   Number of herds/animals found to be infected during year as percentage of the herds/animals tested.

(b)   Expenditure on reactors less receipts from sale of reactors, veterinary fees, tuberculin and haulier payments, other, excluding administration costs.

Source: Department of Agriculture Northern Ireland.

every 6 months and herds in areas in which there is a relatively high level of disease come in for frequent testing. Herds in which there are reactors are tested every 2 months until it is considered safe to lift restrictions. Movement permits are now necessary. These are completed by the herdowners themselves from numbered books of blank forms. The permits are returned to the District Offices after each movement, for validation. The permit system enables checkback on movement of all infected animals. The validation of permits is a laborious and costly process but it is considered necessary for the control of the disease.

Comparison of Costs in the Republic with Those in Northern Ireland

Variable costs (the costs given in Table 7) expressed as percentages of cattle and milk outputs at farm level for the years 1980 to 1984 are given in Table 9 where they are compared with similar figures from Northern Ireland. These figures show that, on average, over the 5 years in question, variable costs in the Republic were about 1.7 per cent of cattle output, 1.91 per cent of milk output and something less than 1 per cent of cattle and milk output combined. The corresponding figures for Northern Ireland where the disease is almost eliminated are about half of these, i.e., 0.81 per cent of cattle output, 1.12 per cent of milk output and 0.47 per cent of milk and cattle combined.

Two points can be made from this table. The first is that variable costs for a full round of testing as a percentage of cattle and milk outputs are much

Table 9: *Variable Costs[a] in Connection with the BTE Scheme as Percentages of Cattle and Milk Outputs in the Irish Republic and in Northern Ireland*

Year	Outputs at Farm Level of:			Variable Costs of BTE Scheme	Variable costs as % of Outputs of:		
	Cattle	Milk	Cattle and Milk		Cattle	Milk	Cattle and Milk
	£m			£m	%		
Irish Republic							
1980	625.8	540.7	1,166.5	10.968	1.75	2.03	0.94
1981	718.2	613.3	1,331.5	12.691	1.77	2.07	0.95
1982	800.6	731.2	1,531.8	13.482	1.68	1.84	0.88
1983	910.6	853.2	1,763.8	15.070	1.65	1.77	0.85
1984	1,040.7	919.3	1,960.0	16.948	1.63	1.84	0.86
Average	—	—	—	—	1.70	1.91	0.88
Northern Ireland							
1980	198.3	132.0	330.3	1.329	0.67	1.01	0.40
1981	220.8	149.2	370.0	1.465	0.66	0.98	0.40
1982	224.4	180.7	405.1	1.928	0.86	1.07	0.48
1983	244.1	201.3	445.4	2.404	0.98	1.19	0.54
1984	283.2	187.9	471.1	2.556	0.90	1.36	0.54
Average	—	—	—	—	0.81	1.12	0.47

(a)   Variable costs are those given in Table 6 for the Irish Republic, namely, net payments for reactors, veterinary surgeons' fees and other costs. Similar items obtained from the Northern Ireland Ministry of Agriculture are included for Northern Ireland.

Sources: Departments of Agriculture, Dublin and Belfast, Statistical Review of Northern Ireland Agriculture 1984, Agricultural Output for 1984, CSO Dublin.

lower in Northern Ireland than in the Republic. The main reason for this is that a full round of testing in the Republic involves up to 1½ tests per animal because of the large number of black spots and the necessity for re-testing at short intervals herds which show reactors. In the North where the disease is at a low level the proportion of animals tested in a round is lower than here, the number of reactors removed is relatively low also and so the relative cost of a round is cheaper. However, the figures would indicate that cost-wise the scheme is not being run as efficiently in the Republic as in Northern Ireland. The matter should be looked at carefully by the Department of Agriculture to see if economies can be brought about.

The second point to be made is that even when the disease is brought down to an acceptably low level in the Republic the eradication costs will not disappear. Round testing will have to take place at least every 2 years, and possibly every year, in order to keep the disease in check while occasional breakdowns will have to be dealt with as they occur. In addition, the fixed costs associated with the District Offices are likely to remain at their present levels into the future. Staff will be required to organise monitoring tests for both brucellosis and tuberculosis. Inspections at meat premises and ports will have to go on and there is no doubt that various other regulations will be introduced. Hence, despite what we do about eliminating tuberculosis in the near future we will not eliminate disease eradication costs.

Chapter 3

THE OPERATION OF THE SCHEME IN RECENT YEARS

The bovine tuberculosis eradication programme is operated through twenty-seven District Veterinary Offices (DVOs) throughout the country, some of them only opened in recent years. A Department of Agriculture/ Department of Finance Review Group which reported on disease eradication schemes in 1983 (Disease Eradication Schemes, 1983) considered that the position in this regard was generally satisfactory except in Cork. This county, which contains almost one million cattle, is serviced from two offices located in Cork City and the Committee Report stated that the disease eradication needs of the county could not be adequately catered for on this basis. It recommended that a District Veterinary Office be provided in West Cork. It also stated that there was a case for a District Office in Longford which currently is served from Roscommon. To date neither of these offices has been provided, though West Cork had the highest incidence of bovine tuberculosis in the State in 1984.

The disease eradication programme (Tuberculosis and Brucellosis) involves approximately 196 permanent veterinary staff, 287 agricultural offices, 623 administrative staff, 148 laboratory staff and 78 others, a total of some 1,332 persons. The agricultural officers' work is to visit farms and factories in connection with the scheme while the administrative staff handle the huge amount of paper work involved. Departmental veterinary officers supervise this scheme and check test animals. In addition there are over 850 private veterinary surgeons involved, with a fairly high proportion of their income coming from this source (Ashton, *et al.*, 1977).

EEC Involvement

When Ireland joined the EEC in 1973 inter-Community trade in bovine animals was (and is) governed by Directive 64/432 EEC and this was a more severe directive than the legislation in use here. Irish records stress incidence of infection measured in a fashion which does not show the complete picture. As explained in Chapter 2 incidence is the proportion of herds or animals in the State which break down in any year as a percentage of the non-restricted herds or animals tested in that year. It takes no account of

41

herds already broken down at the beginning of the year or of supposedly clear herds in which animals with lesions are found at slaughter. Under the EEC rules, herds restricted at the beginning of the year which produce a reactor during the year must be included as well as attested herds which produce a clinical case of tuberculosis during the year (as found at slaughter-houses). The EEC definition is known as herd *Prevalence*. It is the number of herds declared infected in any period as a percentage of the total number of herds in the State.

An Interdepartmental study group which reported in February 1978 (Bovine Tuberculosis Eradication, 1978) stated that incidence of herd infection as calculated by the Department of Agriculture had increased since 1965 from 3.88 to 7.5 per cent and if the EEC definition of prevalence were used 13 per cent of herds would be infected in 1977.

The group further stated that it is obvious from the disease incidence figures (which are given in Table 3) that present eradication methods will not achieve the requisite reduction in the foreseeable future. Indeed, the group doubted that a level of 0.2 per cent of herds infected (as aimed at by the EEC) could be achieved at all unless the eradication programme was considerably overhauled. It said that there has been a lack of commitment on the part of:

(a) herdowners who have not looked on the disease as a serious threat either to their individual livelihood or health or to the economic welfare of the country;

(b) veterinary practitioners, who in general do not seem to have been seriously concerned about getting rid of the disease in the shortest possible time; and

(c) the State because it has not regarded eradication as an absolute priority. It has not outlined a full programme; and has not specified time-bounded attainable targets. It has not always, in practice, demanded absolute co-operation by all parties involved (where insistence might prove unpalatable in the short term).

The Report went on to state that the attitudes of all three sectors would have to change in order to reduce the incidence inside the next few years to the level necessary to ensure that all this country's cattle, beef and dairy products would have access to EEC markets in the years ahead. Unfortunately this reduction in incidence has not yet been attained, 8 years later on.

Trading Considerations

Under the EEC Directive (64/432/EEC) bovine animals for breeding or for milk or meat production may be traded to other Member States only if they originate from officially tuberculosis free herds. In addition if they are over 6 weeks old they must pass a pre-export test (using only the single bovine tuberculin test as distinct from this country's "comparative" test which involves the use of both bovine and avian tuberculins) within 30 days prior to export. At the time of joining the EEC there were no official tuberculosis free herds in Ireland which accorded with the EEC directive. However, Ireland was allowed, under the Treaty of Accession, to use its own method of declaring a herd officially free, but all bovine animals over 6 weeks of age exported to any other Community State must pass the pre-import single tuberculin test described in Chapter 1.

The Accelerated EEC Plan

In 1978 under EEC Directive 77/391 a 3-year accelerated programme for the eradication of bovine tuberculosis and brucellosis was approved by the Commission for Ireland, as well as for France and Italy. In consequence, Ireland qualified for recoupment towards the cost of eradication as follows:

	£'000
1978	1,013
1979	2,613
1980	3,360
1981	2,560

The basis of the Irish plan for the accelerated eradication of tuberculosis was:

(1)   increase in the level of compensation paid to farmers
(2)   special checks in high incidence areas
(3)   provision of proper on-farm handling and isolation facilities
(4)   imposition of a pre-movement tuberculin test.

Special check tests were organised in areas which had demonstrated a high incidence in the previous round of annual testing and also reactor herds were given a special test 6 months after they had gone clear. Provision of proper handling and isolation facilities for animals on farms was made a condition for obtaining reactor grants and for the recognition of any new herds under the Department of Agriculture schemes. From the date of the commencement of the accelerated scheme all bovine animals over 6 weeks of age moved from officially free herds, except those for immediate slaughter, were subject to a pre-movement tuberculin test within 30 days of movement.

Reporting on the accelerated scheme in October 1981 the EEC Commission said:

The bovine tuberculosis scheme is in its 27th year; during the greater part of that time all bovine animals in all Irish herds have been subjected to at least one test every year. Each year between 25,000 and 50,000 animals are removed as reactors. Yet since 1965 there has been no change in the bovine tuberculosis situation in Ireland. (Quoted in Interdepartmental Report — Disease Eradication Schemes, 1983)

In 1982 at the end of the accelerated programme the incidence of the disease in herds was 2.8 per cent, exactly the same as in 1966, and the incidence of the disease in animals from officially free herds as evidenced by lesions in slaughtered animals at export-registered premises had shown little change over the years.

The Commission went on to state that it could not be concluded that the lack of progress with the elimination of the disease was due to lack of finance, but rather to the fundamental fact that two-thirds of the reactors are being missed at annual round tests. In arriving at this conclusion the Commission cited the fact that when the Department engaged a task force of 50 temporary veterinary officers in the early 1970s the task force working on a random sample of about 18 per cent of the national herd found approximately three times as many reactors as the regular veterinary practitioners (Commission of the European Communities, 1981, p. 35).

Commenting on the EEC Commission Report, the 1983 Interdepartmental Review Group stated that:

the report lacked objectivity, was selective in its argumentation and accepted as fact what were merely points of view. Though the report did not say so, there are serious doubts about the randomness of the sample. Nevertheless, the basic underlying message — that progress towards bovine tuberculosis eradication had been unsatisfactory — could not be contested (Disease Eradication Schemes (1983)).

In contrast to Ireland the accelerated schemes in France and Italy were deemed to be successful. In its Report on France at the end of the scheme the EEC Commission stated that Bovine Tuberculosis had reached a low level in France but that it would be necessary to implement specific measures in certain areas in order to further reduce the prevalence of the disease. The proportion of animals with TB lesions discovered at routine slaughter of non-reactor animals during post mortem inspection declined from 0.17 per cent in 1977 to 0.12 per cent in 1980. The incidence of herd infection in 1980 was 1.1 per cent which was slightly above the incidence of 1.0 per cent aimed at (Commission of European Communities, *op. cit.*, p. 31). However, almost 18,000 reactors were discovered in France in 1984 (see Table 2).

In regard to the accelerated scheme in Italy the EEC Commission Report stated that eradication of bovine tuberculosis is proceeding with success (*ibid.*, p. 38). However, as shown in Table 2, Italy has still some way to go before the disease is totally eradicated.

Nomination of Testers

Under Council regulation No. 1055/81 of 21 April 1981 the EEC Council of Ministers, as part of a package of aids to Irish farmers, authorised the introduction of a free pre-movement testing scheme. Under this scheme which was to operate for two years from April 1981, the Irish exchequer was to meet the cost of pre-movement testing for both bovine tuberculosis and brucellosis (which was at the time, and still is, paid for by the herdowners). The EEC was to refund 50 per cent of the cost subject to recoupment being in respect of not more than 1 million cattle per annum and subject to a total reimbursement over the 2 year period of not more than 6 million ECUs (about £4m.). Because of the difficult exchequer situation the scheme was never implemented. If this scheme had been implemented the EEC made it a specific condition that the Department of Agriculture would have the sole right to nominate the private veterinarians who would carry out testing under the scheme.

Though the Department did not adopt Council regulation 1055/81 it did attempt to establish the principle that it (the Department) and not the farmers would have the right to nominate the private veterinarians to do the testing. This development was opposed by the Veterinary Union and culminated in a strike which lasted for about 7 months, and during which only a minimum of testing was done by Department veterinarians. This strike was settled in May 1985 and the 1985/86 round of testing commenced on 3 June 1985. Under the strike settlement, the operation of the scheme was tightened up considerably.

Prior to the 1985 round, veterinary surgeons who had not completed their round of testing by a given date were usually given an extension of time by the DVOs. It is now considered that this was a very undesirable practice which should never have been allowed. Under the revised rules all testing (whether it be round or check testing) issued to a veterinary surgeon must have indicated thereon the final date by which the testing in question is to be completed and this date must be rigidly enforced. No Senior Veterinary Inspector (SVI) has discretion to extend a cut-off date. Testing which has not been completed within the set period must be reallocated. The Department's circular on the matter says:

(1) Testing being reallocated should not be offered to a veterinary surgeon in the practice which failed to carry out the testing on time unless there are compelling reasons for doing so.

(2) Testing allocated to a veterinary surgeon must be completed (and not merely commenced) by the end of the specified testing period.

(3) Under the agreement between the Department and the veterinary union, in so far as monitoring testing is concerned (ordinary round testing) each veterinary practice was offered in 1985 the testing of those herds which that practice tested under the 1983 round of testing updated to take account of developments between then and the end of 1984. All forms of check testing were, however, allocated at the total discretion of the SVI. What this amounts to is that each practice had to be offered one test (tuberculosis and brucellosis) of each herd which that practice tested in 1983 updated to take account of farmer nominations up to the end of 1984) but it had not to be offered any additional testing of these herds which proved necessary.

(4) Such allocation of testing under the 1986 round of testing will be influenced by performance (delivery of testing on time) in 1985. Every DVO will be expected to maintain a performance folder on each veterinary surgeon testing cattle under the programme in the area. Routine reports on supervision of a veterinary surgeon's testing will be kept on these files. Every supervision of a veterinary surgeon must be the subject of a written report.

(5) Any veterinary surgeon may decline testing offered to him/her. If, however, a surgeon undertakes to carry out testing within a stated period, he/she will be expected to honour his/her commitment. If a veterinary surgeon fails to do so he/she will be penalised when testing is being allocated in 1986 unless a valid reason for failure is forthcoming.

(6) If a herdowner whose herd is listed for testing postpones testing the VS may arrange by telephone for the substitution of another herd. If the volume of cancellations notified by a VS to a DVO is very great and repeated further testing will not be issued to him/her and the matter will be reported to Head Office.

(7) Where a farmer postpones testing twice for no valid reason, the herd will be restricted and the matter referred to the

Gardai if the herdowner persists in being uncooperative.

(8) It can be expected that in some few cases a herdowner may decline to have his herd tested by a particular practitioner. Such cases are to be resolved by selecting an alternative practitioner or inspector, but not one chosen by the herdowner.

(9) Where a veterinary surgeon retires or dies, any lien which he/she may have on the monitoring round between the Veterinary Union and the Department ceases to exist at that point. In the case of a multiple practice the practice loses its lien on a number of herds equivalent to the number of herds divided by the number of principals in the practice. From that point on, an SVI may allocate the monitor testing of those herds at his/her total discretion and a veterinary surgeon who buys out the practice has no lien on the herds. It is to be anticipated however, that in many instances the SVI may continue to allocate monitor testing of a number of the herds in question to a veterinary surgeon in the practice.

(10) Fees for testing shall be paid to the veterinary surgeon (and not the practice) who has carried out the test unless written instructions to the contrary are received from the veterinary surgeon.

(11) Each veterinary surgeon testing cattle under the programme must be supervised at least once during each round of testing. A copy of the report of the supervisory officer will be filed in the veterinary officer's performance folder (see Section 4 above).

(12) For the future, no veterinary surgeon (whether in private practice or on the Department's staff) is permitted to test his/her own herd or the herd of a parent or son/daughter.

The result of those changes has been quite dramatic as far as punctuality of testing is concerned. Testing provides a major portion of most veterinary surgeons' incomes and they do not wish to have that income jeopardised by failure to do their testing in time. The new rules also gave the SVI the opportunity of curtailing the activities of unsatisfactory testers and of allowing young veterinary surgeons to become established. As shown later, however, the establishment of young veterinary surgeons has not materialised by this route.

The rules provide for supervision of "testers" at least once during each round of testing. This rule has always been in operation but it is hoped that it will be applied more vigorously in future than in the past. The most difficult supervision problem occurs with careless "testers" who perform adequately during the inspection period but who revert to their normal methods when the inspector is not there. For these, and indeed for all "testers", independent checks by Department Inspectors are necessary to determine if reactors are being missed in round tests. Indeed, in all areas where the disease is persistent, successive tests should alternate between the normal testers and Departmental Inspectors. This can be accomplished more easily under the new rules than in the past. Whether it is introduced and leads to an acceleration in the eradication of the disease remains to be seen.

High Risk Areas

One of the problems with the eradication programme is the continuing prevalence of high risk areas where the disease seems to be almost endemic. Reporting on the situation in 1982, Mr R.G. Cullen, Director of Veterinary Services in the Department of Agriculture (Cullen, 1982) said that the disease picture is not a uniform one. Tuberculosis is still at its lowest in the general area north of a line drawn from Drogheda to Galway City, but even inside that area a large amount of disease is focused in districts such as Milford in Co. Donegal, Central Sligo, South East Mayo which includes parts of Roscommon and Galway. He said the worst counties were in the South East of the country — Waterford, Kilkenny, Carlow and Wexford with North Kerry pretty bad also. In 1977 herd incidence in these counties varied between 9 and 17 per cent, the latter figure representing Kilkenny, then the worst county in Ireland. However, as a result of the EEC Acceleration Programme the herd incidence in these counties was reduced to between 2 and 4 per cent. In more recent years, Cork South West, Longford, Westmeath, Clare and Tipperary North have had serious problems with the disease seeming to run rapidly from farm to farm. The figures in Table 10 giving the herd incidence on a county basis for some recent years, show that the rate is very variable. In 1984 the counties with the highest incidence were Offaly (5.0), Wicklow West (4.54), Clare (4.29), Tipperary North (4.24), and Cork South West (4.00).[6] These are average figures for the counties, but in most counties there are clear areas as well as high pockets of infection which are most difficult to clear.

In his paper, Cullen (*ibid.*) made reference to outbreaks occurring regularly in clusters of 6 to 10 herds, all of which are sometimes up one lane with cattle from different herds continually mixing. He made the following additional points:

---

6. Though the level of these figures must be taken with some caution, they do show that the rate of infection is very variable throughout the country.

Table 10: *Bovine Tuberculosis Herd Incidence by County 1980-1984*

County	No. of Herds 1984	Herd Incidence %				
		1980	1981	1982	1983	1984
Carlow	2,073	3.03	2.08	3.47	3.49	2.39
Cavan	8,104	1.53	1.73	1.29	1.58	1.70
Clare	9,295	2.73	2.63	4.74	3.83	4.29
Cork N/E } Cork S/W }	19,932	6.49	4.25	5.02	2.68 / 4.84	2.67 / 4.00
Donegal	12,221	0.76	0.59	0.93	2.67	0.56
Dublin	1,055	2.32	1.42	1.72	0.73	1.69
Galway	18,257	2.12	2.14	3.20	3.19	2.08
Kerry	12,630	3.69	2.11	2.25	3.06	1.43
Kildare	3,464	3.80	2.69	4.13	2.74	2.95
Kilkenny	4,709	4.30	2.96	3.09	2.51	3.76
Laois	4,399	2.88	2.59	4.51	2.49	3.17
Leitrim	5,463	1.12	0.43	0.90	1.86	1.31
Limerick	9,533	2.43	2.15	2.30	2.58	1.59
Longford	3,879	3.61	3.04	3.52	3.82	3.36
Louth	12,780	2.67	1.66	1.68	1.41	1.20
Mayo	17,407	0.83	0.82	0.79	—	0.75
Meath	6,388	3.53	2.60	2.34	2.17	2.60
Monaghan	6,059	3.62	2.30	2.24	2.14	2.13
Offaly	4,563	3.34	2.90	3.90	3.91	5.00
Roscommon	9,222	1.30	1.15	2.33	4.08	2.52
Sligo	6,629	0.74	0.65	0.68	0.89	0.37
Tipperary North } Tipperary South }	11,317	3.79	2.40	3.24	4.32	4.24 / 2.59
Waterford	3,540	3.32	2.52	3.74	2.63	1.88
Westmeath	4,568	4.88	3.49	5.47	4.37	3.64
Wexford	5,267	3.32	2.11	2.53	2.76	1.77
Wicklow East } Wicklow West }	2,734	3.65	2.76	3.58	2.24 / 2.10	3.35 / 4.54
Total	195,488	2.94	2.11	2.76	3.16	2.24

Source: Department of Agriculture.

(1) Many of the herds which had the disease in the past 5 years are going down again — *continuing infection*

(2) Neighbouring herds to these are also going down — *lateral spread*

(3) Cattle are spreading the disease to other cattle simply by movement. This can happen with cattle moving (a) legally on

a 30-day certificate and calves under 6 weeks of age; (b) illegally such as calves and other cattle from a diseased herd; (c) cattle mixing because of commonage, bad fencing, shared crushes and even going to a bull in a diseased herd, or vice versa.

It also happens with movement of cattle to rented land some miles away or to fragmented parts of farms. He went on to say that the disease was being spread from animal to animal across fences and gates when neighbouring cattle nose each other. Nosing was very noticeable at watering places, along banks of rivers, lakes and streams where cattle congregate in hot weather and where only a single strand of wire often separates healthy and diseased stock. Good fencing is absolutely essential and double fencing using an electric fence is better.

Not all of the veterinary profession would agree that cattle contact is the main source of infection. A recent report of a meeting of the Connacht Clinical Society published in the *Irish Veterinary News* (December 1985) quoted a number of speakers as saying that cattle were also becoming infected with tuberculosis from some other source, badgers being mentioned as the main culprits. The Irish evidence for this view is, however, not very conclusive, but research on the problem is being carried out, both by the Department of Agriculture and the Veterinary College. The Department, while not ruling out the role of the badger in spreading the disease, gives it a low priority. They claim on the basis of their evidence to date that cattle contact is by far the greatest cause at the present time, particularly contact when animals are under stressful conditions due to poor feeding, wet lying conditions, travelling to marts, etc. (Personal communication with J. Noonan, Deputy Director of Veterinary Services in the Department of Agriculture). When the incidence of the disease becomes lower, of course, badgers are likely to be a potent source of infection in certain instances, as is presumed to be the case in Southwest England (see Chapter 1). At that time, also, deer, goats and even humans may be important sources of infection.

Chapter 4

DEFECTS IN THE EXISTING BTE SCHEME

Numerous reports on the eradication of bovine tuberculosis in Ireland, some of which have been referred to in earlier chapters, have been prepared over the years. Practically all have referred to defects in the scheme and have made suggestions for improvement. In this chapter I quote from three fairly recent reports which cover most of the points that can be mentioned. My own comments on the more important of these points are made in the next chapter. The reports in question are:

(1) The 1983 Interdepartmental Committee Report (Disease Eradication Scheme, 1983)
(2) The 1984 Conjoint Report by all the veterinary groups (The Eradication of Tuberculosis in Cattle, 1984)
(3) A Report giving the views and recommendations of
    (a) The Irish Farmers' Associations (IFA) (1982)
    (b) The Irish Veterinary Union (1982) and
    (c) The Irish Veterinary Association (1979) entitled Eradication of Tuberculosis in Cattle (January 1982).

As a general point the Interdepartmental Committee said that the strategy adopted in the early 1950s of commencing bovine TB clearance measures in the north west and gradually extending these measures to the rest of the country was ill conceived. The approach was dictated by the trading situation of the time, by the need to minimise the impact on the cattle trade and dairy industry and by the pressure for rapid results. This strategy failed to take due account of the traditional pattern of cattle movement in this country — from the southern dairying (calf producing) areas to the western counties for rearing and then to the fattening areas of the midlands and east for finishing. Experience has shown that, with movement of young stock from the south (where TB incidence has remained relatively high) cleared areas in other parts of the State have become reinfected and the disease has cropped up in areas where tuberculosis had not been recorded for many years.

The implication here is that the west and midland regions of the country are still being reinfected from the south and the group recommended the setting up of special status zones in the southern production counties from which young stock would move to the west and midlands.

Nomination of Testers

Since the scheme was introduced in 1954 each herdowner was allowed to nominate the private veterinary surgeon who would test his cattle. Only in the case of retesting of reactor herds or inconclusives and check testing of areas where disease incidence was high did the Department of Agriculture reserve the right to nominate the veterinarian who would do the testing. The Interdepartmental Report stated that there is ample evidence that this close relationship between the herdowner and the practitioner who normally did his testing was damaging to the BTE programme. It resulted in pressure on the practitioner to give cattle a "soft" test and there have been numerous examples of a herdowner transferring his testing to another veterinarian after his normal practitioner had disclosed a reactor in the herd.

The Report said that this system was fair neither to the conscientious practitioner nor to the taxpayer. It resulted in

(a)   diseased animals remaining in herds
(b)   disease being spread by animals which should have been removed as reactors and
(c)   a general dilution of the Department of Agriculture's control of the scheme.

As stated in the last chapter the EEC Commission recognised this flaw. It insisted that under the free pre-movement scheme (which was not implemented) the Department should have the right to nominate the veterinarian doing the testing. The Commission was adamant that Ireland's extended acceleration plan would not be approved unless it provided for "special status zones" in which successive tests would alternate between the veterinarians who would normally do the testing and an official Department-nominated veterinarian. This change was put into operation in Kerry from 30 June 1983. Other special status zones were not developed, the Department having taken the view that the intensive testing carried out in 1985/86 and foreseen for the remainder of the government's three year programme (but not carried out) afforded an opportunity for progress at least comparable to that expected from special status zones.

Lack of Commitment by All Concerned

In 1965 when the Minister declared the country to be fully attested there were supposed to be good economic and trading reasons for this step. With hindsight, however, the 1965 decision must be seen as unfortunate. It is now clear that the disease was very far from being eradicated at that time and that major problems were ahead. The decision gave rise to a sense of false security among farmers and to bewilderment and frustration when the disease incidence rose significantly in the following decade. This led to a loss of confidence in the BTE scheme and the problem remains to the present day. The fact that the scheme has now been in operation for more than 30 years without ultimate success being in sight has led to a "tiredness", lack of commitment, and almost a resigned acceptedness by some herdowners that bovine tuberculosis will always be with us despite heavy expenditure on eradication every year.

The Interdepartmental group recommended the introduction of an intensive advertising and publicity campaign to bring home to farmers the cost of bovine tuberculosis and the benefits which would accrue from rapid eradication of the disease. The group also recommended vigorous and consistent enforcement of the disease regulations. In order to implement these recommendations the farming organisations have held meetings all over the country pointing out the heavy losses incurred as a result of herd breakdowns and urging their members to take the recommended precautions and obey the eradication rules.

High Volume of Cattle Movement

Ireland is unique within the Community as regards the volume and frequency of cattle movement, estimated at 6 million movements per annum (Store Cattle Study Group Report (1968) and Report by Irish Fresh Meat Exporters' Society (A Strategy for the Development of Irish Cattle and Beef Industry 1981)). This movement creates obvious problems for disease eradication and it is impossible to do much about it. It has been suggested by the IVA and the IFA that cattle should only be moved under movement permits, as in Britain and Northern Ireland. To a certain extent this is happening already. All animals, other than calves under 6 weeks of age, offered for sale must have a pre-movement test which is valid for 60 days at the present time.[7] The results of this test are written on the animal's registration card and so the card becomes in fact a movement permit valid for 60 days which can be examined at any time by authorised officers. Animals moving along the road from one part of a farm to another do not require pre-movement tests. Neither do animals going directly from a farm for immediate slaughter or for export to countries outside the EEC. The latter can move on a "valid" identity card which is the registration card showing that the animal was tested within the past 18 months. If an animal is not tested within 18 months the identity card is not valid for movement, and the farmer may be required to have a test carried out.

7. A 30-day test is still required for intra Community trade.

The IFA says that the present system is open to widespread abuse by farmers and cattle dealers, particularly in relation to the direct movement for slaughter, and they claim that these animals should only move on permit also. They do stipulate, however, that the introduction of the permit system should coincide with the introduction of free pre-movement testing. This puts the matter in a slightly different perspective. The Department is loathe to have free pre-movement testing as it would be very costly to the State.

One of the purposes of a movement permit system is to enable animal movement to be traced in cases where outbreaks of the disease occur. The present system does not enable this to be done. An animal could move to several farms in 60 days and could have several owners, making trace-back impossible. In order to facilitate trace-back it is now generally agreed that particulars of all animals in the State should be recorded on computers and every movement recorded. A system of computer registration is currently being introduced here and when completed the permit system will be initiated in an effort to record and trace all cattle movements. The computer records can also be used to ensure that all animals are presented for testing at a test. The veterinary organisations claim that many animals are not being presented for testing in the first instance, and that is the reason why a very high number of lesion-positive carcases show up at slaughterhouses. Animals coming in and out of herds on legal or illegal movement are gone before the test while others on out farms or on 11 months land are never presented for testing.

Illegal Movement

The Conjoint Report expresses concern at the extent to which cattle and calves in particular appear to be moved from restricted holdings. It says that the difficulties associated with the control of this practice are recognised but these difficulties are not in themselves acceptable as an excuse for failure to control this established source of infection for other herds. It recommended that quarantine procedures be instituted on all restricted holdings so as to ensure against the illegal movement of cattle of any age off such premises. It said that if these measures impose undue hardship on landowners due to lack of fodder or suitable housing for young stock, funds should be made available to meet such contingencies.

Defective Testing

The Inderdepartmental group stated that defective or careless testing has undoubtedly contributed to the lack of progress. They attributed this to a number of factors:

(a)   the farmer/veterinary relationship which puts heavy pressure on the veterinary practitioner to carry out a "soft" test

(b)   the lack of motivation among veterinary practitioners resulting from the fact that the scheme has been in operation for so long without much success and

(c)   culpable negligence on the part of some veterinarians.

As was noted in the previous chapter testing by private practitioners is likely, in future, to be supervised on a regular and systematic basis and this should achieve an improvement in testing standards.

Transport Vehicles

The existing legislation in relation to the cleanliness of vehicles used to transport cattle and other farm animals has, in the opinion of many observers, proved to be totally ineffective. There is no organised system for the inspection or disinfection of such vehicles even those which are used to transport infected reactor cattle to Department of Agriculture supervised slaughtering premises. The Interdepartmental study group recommended that more effective legislation to deal with the problem of "dirty" lorries should be introduced as a matter of urgency. It stated that consideration might be given to introducing a system on the lines of that operating in France where a vehicle transporting animals must display a dated disc issued by the police which certifies that the vehicle was inspected and was found to be clean when the animals were loaded.

Collection of Reactors and Cattle Dealer Activities

Up to 1976 the Department of Agriculture purchased reactors at negotiated prices and arranged for collection and delivery to slaughtering plants. Since 1976 herdowners themselves have had to arrange for the delivery of reactors to approved slaughter premises, and in addition to the factory price, herd-owners qualified for reactor payments from the Department. This change was made at the request of the farming organisations who now probably regret the decision. The Department compensation for certain classes of cattle such as cows is not very high and reactor cattle are heavily downgraded in price at the factories. (For scale of payments for reactors and herd depopulation see Appendix B).

In most instances reactors are now collected by dealers and hauliers for delivery to slaughter premises. The Interdepartmental Report says that this development amounts to an abandonment of official control of the movement of known infected animals. There is no way of ensuring that lorries are disinfected after transport and since infected animals are often held illegally on dealers' lands until a full load is obtained there is always the danger that the reactor cattle will infect healthy animals on these or neighbouring lands.

Indeed many cattle dealers (and farmers) put trading considerations before animal health or disease eradication. As a consequence healthy cattle come into contact with infected animals. Dealers are required to register with the Department and to keep records of all purchases and sales. Their premises are subject to twice yearly testing but their stock may be at a very low level when a test is made. The Interdepartmental group recommended that for the future all testing of cattle dealers' herds should be carried out by Departmental veterinary staff and suggested that testing should be timed to coincide with periods when stocking levels can be expected to be high.

Re-Testing of Reactor and Inconclusive Herds

A reactor herd should be re-tested as soon as is deemed necessary (usually 60 days) after cleansing and disinfection of premises have been completed following disposal of reactors. In practice it can happen for periods much longer than 60 days to elapse before re-testing despite the full co-operation the herdowner. This results in herds being restricted for unnecessarily long periods. Tighter organisation at District Veterinary Office level should, however, resolve this problem.

Depopulation of Herds and Additional Funding

A very important area which needs to be tackled, is the total depopulation of herds. Bovine tuberculosis is very much akin to human tuberculosis. It becomes endemic in a herd and often cannot be got rid of without eliminating the entire herd. In the past, this often created very serious social conditions for dairy farmers in particular, because the depopulation grant available up to May 1986 was barely sufficient to restock the farm and left nothing for current income. It also placed a great strain on the Department Inspectors as well as on the local veterinary practitioners. These officials were usually loathe to order complete depopulation because it would often mean bankruptcy for the herdowner. In many cases, therefore, depopulation was not recommended even though the presence was suspected of undisclosed carriers which showed no reaction, and these continued to infect healthy animals giving rise to chronic conditions.

The 1983 Interdepartmental Report said that there are possibly 400 chronically affected herds in the State which constitute a continuing infection risk for neighbouring herds and a constant drain on the exchequer. It would be more economic from the point of view of the herdowners and the exchequer to depopulate these herds and budgetary provision should be made for this.

In the recent White Paper *Building on Reality* (1984) the Government said that substantial additional funding is being set aside for disease eradication including new special assistance for herd depopulation. There will also be an increase in the bovine disease eradication levy for one year from November 1984 to yield an additional £7 million in 1985.

The extra funding for depopulation has now been made available (see Appendix B) and there should, therefore, be no hesitation about depopulating herds where there is endemic infection.

Epidemiology

The 1983 Interdepartmental group stated that epidemiology (the study of disease and its spread) had necessarily to be low on the Department's list of priorities while bovine tuberculosis was widespread. In 1983 when 5,000 to 6,000 herds were restricted, the tracing of the source of infection in these and all new breakdowns would be a most demanding task. The group considered, however, that henceforth no effort should be spared to carry out a trace-back exercise in all instances through the introduction of computerisation.

Financial Contribution from Farming Sector

The Interdepartmental group concluded that the final elimination of disease must be seen as a long-term objective and some members recommended a financial contribution from the farming sector, this sector being the main beneficiary of the disease eradication. Such a contribution is now being collected in the form of levies of 0.6p per gallon of milk sold and £3.80 per bovine animal killed at export slaughter premises or exported alive. No charge is made on animals slaughtered for the home market. Some farmers interviewed in connection with this study have argued that these levies are too remote and do little to hasten eradication. They say that the levies should be more closely related to outbreaks but they were rather vague as to how this should be done.

National Manager and Executive Office

The Conjoint Report states bluntly that the scheme is not being properly managed by the Department. It says that

(1)   there is a lack of direction in the overall programme attributable to the absence of a national manager and identifiable operational targets;

(2)   there is failure to enforce the existing legislation regarding in particular
(a) the movement of cattle

  (b) the performance of the tuberculin test and the conditions under which the test has to be conducted on many holdings and

  (c) the control of contaminated materials

(3) There is failure to utilise to the fullest possible extent the resources which are available or are claimed to be available, viz.

  (a) complete surveillance and data retrieval regarding tuberculosis in cattle slaughtered at all domestic and export premises

  (b) surveillance by means of the pre-movement tuberculin test of cattle destined for export to third countries and

  (c) the investigative and control procedures including quarantine and disinfection of premises; and

(4) a misconception on the part of the national funding agencies that the Bovine Tuberculosis Eradication Scheme is solely an animal health matter without due regard to the public health aspects of the disease or to the service which the eradication programme provides to the dairy, meat and cattle industries.

These are very strong criticisms but the Report goes further and recommends that the operation of the scheme be taken out of the Department and set up as an Executive Office with a National Manager.[8] These criticisms and the idea of a National Manager are discussed in the next chapter.

Animal Identification

It was stated in the Conjoint Report that the official animal identity eartag currently in use was unsatisfactory in many ways. Since that Report was written an adapted Herberholz tag has been brought into use which is regarded as being satisfactory. The Conjoint Report also suggested that herd-owners be given legal responsibility for tagging their own cattle for official identification purposes.

Disinfection of Premises

The veterinary profession, as might be expected, places a good deal of emphasis on

(a) the cleaning and disinfection of infected premises, including vehicles,

(b) the storage and disinfection of slurries and manures on infected holdings, and

8. For a discussion on the structure of an Executive Office see the 1985 White Paper on the Public Service, Serving the Country Better, Department of Public Service.

(c)   the use of grassland likely to be contaminated by M. bovis.

The Conjoint Report recommends that research be undertaken or extended into the efficiency of approved disinfectants and of the approved cleaning and disinfection procedures in the context of modern production systems. The veterinary profession also recommends expenditure on research for the development of a serological test.

Severe Interpretation of Test

On farms where the disease persists the severe interpretation of the test is used to ensure that all reactors are removed, whereas on other farms the standard interpretation is used. The IFA recommend that a uniform system of interpretation should apply for all internal movement of cattle. They say that "the operation of two interpretations in TB testing is unwise and rightly or wrongly the impression is created that some level of disease is tolerable in the national herd". The Department has different views in this regard. It claims that if the severe interpretation only were used in such or indeed any test an unacceptably large number of non-infected animals would be removed. The use of the standard interpretation with an inconclusive category allows some flexibility in testing, particularly in herds and in parts of the country where there are very low rates of infection.

B.N. MacClancy, Director of the Veterinary Research Laboratory, Abbotstown, in an unpublished report (MacClancy, 1962-63) says that during the course of experiments carried out in this country in co-operation with the British Ministry of Agriculture, Fisheries and Food, some measure of the reliability of the single intradermal comparative test, as performed by Irish practitioners in the course of the BTE scheme, was obtained. Of 510 cow reactors subjected to careful post-mortem examination, tuberculosis lesions were found in 395 (77.5 per cent) while the remaining 22.5 per cent were classed as non-visible lesion (NVL) reactors. A considerable proportion of those NVL reactors was uninfected (false positives) and therefore an index of the severity of the test. If the severe interpretation had been used a much higher proportion of false positives would have been discovered which would have been very wasteful. O'Reilly (1969a) says that as long as false positive reactors remain a small percentage of the total animals tested, the economic burden can be borne, but when the proportion gets high, as would be the case if the severe test were applied to all herds, herdowners and the State would be subject to considerable loss. Hence, in his opinion, the practice of applying the standard interpretation to herds which are suspected to be clear can hardly be faulted. As stated in Chapter 1 the use of the severe interpretation in infected herds is to ensure that, as far as possible, all infected animals are identified in such herds even if some healthy animals are removed as reactors.

The loss from doing this is small, since only about 5,000 herds are involved at any one time compared with about 190,000 clear herds.

In view of the above discussion it is somewhat surprising to see the Farmers' Association agreeing to a suggestion that the severe interpretation be applied for all pre-movement tests (Eradication of Tuberculosis, 1982, p. 4). The data in Table 7 would seem to indicate that there are already a fairly large number of non-infected animals being removed as reactors at a high cost to herd-owners. If the severe interpretation were to be applied for movement testing many more non-infected cattle would be removed and would give the impression that the disease is more widespread than, in fact, it is.

Chapter 5

CONCLUSIONS AND RECOMMENDATIONS

Having reviewed the various suggestions for improvement put forward by the different bodies I now turn to examine the key elements in these suggestions and make some further points.

Cattle Movement, Contact and Trace-Back

In this paper there has been reference to cattle movement and contact as major problems in the BTE programme particularly when animals are in stressful conditions. Movement, of course, cannot be stopped in Ireland. It is part of our economic structure. Herdowners depend on cattle sales for cash flow, towns depend on cattle marts for much of their business; farmers in the west and midlands depend on the dairy farmers in the south for their supply of calves, while large numbers of people make their living from trading in and transporting stock. Cattle movement must, therefore, go on in our peculiar pastoral climate. What must be done, however, is to control and monitor the movement. The control and monitoring of up to 6 million movements a year is, however, a most formidable and costly undertaking.

It was suggested in the previous chapter that special status zones should be set up in the southern calf-producing counties from which young stock would move to the west and midlands. It would be very difficult to ensure that calves from these zones only moved northwards. Where would the calves from the non-special status zones in the south go? If a scheme such as this were to be brought into operation it would be better to start area clearance all over again and systematically clear the whole country starting with the southern counties and moving northwards in line with calf movements. This may eventually have to be done, but other means should be tried first as supervision would be very costly.

Another idea suggested was the issue of movement permits. This also is a difficult and costly operation. Having to obtain a permit for every movement is very restrictive. In Northern Ireland the farmer is allowed to write his own permit which is validated later on its return to the District Office. Such a system could work here if every herdowner were issued with a book of consecutively numbered dockets which could be checked from time to

61

time by inspectors. A docket should be written out for every movement and returned to the DVO the next day. Heavy fines should be imposed for movement without completed dockets. The validation of dockets in the veterinary office is, however, very time consuming and to do it manually would require considerable resources. Cattle records must, therefore, be computerised and even then the issue of permits to herdowners as required will be a costly operation. It must be done, however, if illegal movement is to be controlled and successful trace-back of infected cattle accomplished. In regard to trace-back an area which requires attention is the post-mortem inspection of animals slaughtered at butchers' premises. Such inspections are not carried out on all animals and until this is done a complete check-back cannot be undertaken.[9] The Department of Agriculture is currently engaged in computerising the cattle records, but a movement permit capability is not envisaged before the end of 1988.

But, of course, monitoring or even control of movement will not prevent the disease spreading to some extent. Movement to marts and sales means contact between cattle, some of which are carrying infection and this inevitably means lateral spread. There is also contact through cattle from different herds meeting on laneways and through nosing across boundary fences. There should, therefore, be greater emphasis by the Department on the need for stock proof boundary fencing in the official advertising and publicity campaigns related to disease control.

Identification of Cattle, Illegal Movement and Other Illegal Practices

The Conjoint Report recommended that quarantine procedures be introduced on all restricted holdings so as to ensure against the illegal movement of cattle of all ages (including calves) off such holdings. What is meant by quarantine in this context is not clear. If it means placing inspectors at farm gates all over the country, it is an impracticable suggestion. The cost of supervising 5,000 farms would be prohibitive and would be ineffective on fragmented holdings since the inspector could not be in two places at the same time.

The problem, however, is serious. There are frequent reports in the newspapers and elsewhere of tag switching on older cattle and illegal movement of calves from restricted holdings. Older cattle cannot easily be moved from locked-up holdings because their registration cards are in the District Office. If these cattle are moved their ear-tags must be switched and corresponding registration cards must be obtained. In the past, tags and cards were usually obtained from butchers' premises which are not subject to regular veterinary

---

9. Proposed new slaughterhouse legislation is designed to cater for this problem.

inspection. The tags from these premises could be opened and re-used.

To overcome the problem of tag switching, the Department has experimented over the years with several types of tag but until recently it has been unable to find one which could not be re-opened and re-closed successfully. The latest version is a light tag suitable for calves which breaks easily if re-opened. This tag may succeed in preventing tag switching, but knowing the ingenuity of herdowners one cannot be too optimistic. We must hope for the best and advocate very heavy fines for those caught switching tags.

Unlike older cattle, animals under 6 weeks of age could easily be moved off restricted holdings because they do not require ear-tags or cards. One way of dealing with this problem would be to require that all calves be tested prior to movement and issued with tags and registration cards.

To insist, however, on a pre-movement test for all calves would be unduly restrictive and costly and would not be effective. O'Reilly (1982) in an internal Departmental memorandum says that the time from which infection occurs in calves until a skin allergy appears varies from 8 to 51 days, with the vast majority reacting to the test 3 to 4 weeks after infection. Since most calves are sold within the first 10 days of life, the test would be negative in practically all cases and would therefore be unlikely to serve any useful purpose.

One way out of the illegal calf movement problem would be to allow herdowners to tag their own calves as suggested in the Conjoint Report. If this system were adopted, no calf should be allowed move to another herd without a numbered ear-tag. All calves could thus be traced back to their herd of origin and there would be a check on movement from restricted herds. It is recommended that this suggestion be adopted. There is, of course, a danger involved in giving out tags to herdowners but if farmers were made accountable for all tags received and fined heavily for missing tags the system would be workable.

In addition to illegal movement there is another illicit practice which is believed to be fairly common. Certain antibiotics can be used to reduce the lumps on the skin of reactor animals and it is claimed that some herdowners use these chemicals to mask reactions. The chemicals in question can be purchased without a prescription at the present time, but putting them on prescription is no help since they can be stored and used later for illicit purposes. This alleged practice should be investigated as a matter of urgency and steps taken to deal with it if it is found to be common.

Nomination of Testers

Since the beginning of the 1985/86 round when the Department succeeded in its demands to have the right to nominate testers, the position in regard to punctuality of testing has improved considerably. Though the rules state that the 1986 round of testing will be allocated at the sole discretion of the DVO, it has turned out that practitioners who performed adequately in 1985 have been allocated the same herds in the 1986 round, namely, their own clients' herds. Under present arrangements where private practitioners are doing the testing, it is impossible for the Department to do otherwise except in the rare cases where veterinary surgeons are found to be doing inadequate work or not doing the testing on time. Hence, practitioners continue, as in the past, to test their own clients' herds and young veterinarians are not being established in practice as had been suggested in Chapter 3.

The only way to get over these problems would be to have all the testing done by Departmental veterinarians. This would mean a huge expansion in the Department's staff and would be very costly if whole-time officers were employed. However, if staff were employed in a part-time capacity and paid on a per test basis, the cost would not be much greater than at present. Private practitioners would have to be employed on such a scheme as there are not sufficient other veterinarians available, but it is unlikely that many would leave their practices for prolonged periods. However, if the disease is not well on the way to being cleared up within the next 3 years, the Department or some other body may have no option except to take over all the testing themselves and seek staff wherever they can be found. Even though this system may be no better than the present one, some changes will have to be made, if there are no improvements, in order to allay public disquiet on the subject. It is estimated that about 230 extra veterinary surgeons would have to be employed and that the payments to these for a full round of testing, including intensive testing of black spots, would be about £13 million in 1985 compared with an actual payment of £11 million veterinary fees in that year.

Reliability of the Test and Defective Testing

The reliability of the test is discussed in Appendix A where it is shown that some controversy has arisen as to its accuracy. The academic veterinarians say it is only 80-85 per cent accurate and less than that in old cows. On the basis of this view the veterinarians imply that it will be difficult if not impossible to eradicate the disease without the aid of a blood test as a back-up for dificult cases.

The Chief Scientific Officer of the Department's Veterinary Research Laboratory, on the other hand, claims that the test is 98 per cent reliable when applied in accordance with the Department's instructions, that it has succeeded in eradicating the disease in other countries and that there is no reason why it should not do the same here if properly administered.

A good blood test as a back-up to the skin test would undoubtedly be a great help, but as stated in Appendix A, the likelihood of developing such a test in the near future is remote, despite heavy expenditure throughout the world on research in this area, both for human and bovine tuberculosis. Every few years there are reports in the literature of a breakthrough being expected, but as Kardjito and Grange (1985) say, "all the tests developed to date have failed miserably in clinical practice". We must therefore rely on the normal skin test and make the best of it regardless of its degree of reliability.

This raises the question of the application of the test. The EEC Report (1981) stated that a large number of reactors were being missed on the round tests, but this was disputed by the Department of Agriculture, whose officials have stated that the trial carried out by the EEC was unscientific and the results thus unreliable. In any case, checking on the reliability of tests is a most difficult area because of the rapidity with which the disease spreads. However, because of public disquiet, the matter should be re-examined. The EEC should be asked to send in a team of outside veterinarians to check test a random sample of herds due for an annual test and to carry out post-mortem examinations on all reactor animals. In this way it may be possible to judge the efficacy of testing and have the matter settled one way or another. The EEC officers should also be asked to check and report on the holding facilities available on farms and to recommend that those with inadequate facilities be restricted until such time as proper facilities are provided.

Lack of Commitment to the Scheme by All Concerned

Most herdowners do their best to obey the rules, but there are many others, some well known to the authorities, who flout the rules continually, either through carelessness, design, or ignorance and are mainly responsible for spreading the disease to clean herds. At one stage a special Garda was assigned to every DVO for the purpose of dealing with breaches of the eradication laws and this system worked well. Due to curtailment of funds the scheme has now been abandoned, but those in charge feel that it should be re-introduced if the disease is to be eradicated. The fact that a uniformed Garda is likely to turn up with a veterinarian to investigate a herd breakdown makes people think twice about their behaviour in relation to the disease. It is suggested that this scheme be re-introduced and that cattle dealers' herds be tested every 6 months.

In regard to the other groups involved, i.e., the veterinary practitioners and the Department Inspectors, there is an impression abroad that there is no great urgency on their part to eliminate the disease. This view is based on an impression that if the disease were eradicated a large number of people would have worked themselves out of employment. It has been shown in Chapter 2 that this is not so for the Departmental Inspectors. Were testing to be substantially reduced the veterinary and other staff at District Offices would be employed in carrying out duties in relation to a wide range of animal health and other welfare matters.

Veterinary practititioners will also be employed for the foreseeable future on these duties, but as some areas of the country get cleared up revenue from testing will be reduced in these places. It is doubtful, however, if this prospect affects the work of the ordinary practitioner. The vast majority of people everywhere do the job they are paid to do, to the best of their abilities and it is likely to be the same among the workers in this scheme. In all organisations and in all countries there are, of course, careless people who do not carry out their duties as well as they should and there are such people among the veterinary practitioners here. These are well known to the authorities and should be kept under constant check. On the whole, however, there is no reason to believe that standards are much worse here than in countries which have eliminated the disease. We are dealing with a very difficult problem for which there is no easy solution, and when things do not come right everybody tends to blame everybody else.

Transport Vehicles

It was stated in the previous chapter that the legislation relating to cleanliness of vehicles used to transport cattle has proved to be totally ineffective and it was suggested that a police disc system, as in France, might be introduced here. The disc issued by the police would certify that the lorry was inspected and found to be clean. This seems to be an impracticable system. Unless he sees a lorry being disinfected a police officer cannot certify that it is clean.

Something must be done in this regard, however, and the best thing would be to ensure that all trucks leaving marts and slaughterhouses are washed and disinfected. Facilities for doing this are mandatory in all such premises but there is no legal requirement that they be used. The law in this regard should be changed so as to ensure that all cattle trucks are disinfected before leaving marts and slaughterhouses and discs issued to drivers when the operation is completed. Spot checks on lorries leaving marts and slaughterhouses should be made by Gardai to see if the vehicles have been washed and lookouts should be kept by Department Inspectors in these premises to see that proper washing is done.

Collection of Reactors

In regard to the collection of reactors, changes in the rules are required as a matter of urgency. Allowing dealers to collect reactors is asking for trouble and the system must be stopped regardless of cost. Reactor cattle should go direct from farm to factory and there should be no intermediate stops as very often happens at present.

It is understood that the Department is looking into this matter and that arrangements are being made with co-operatives to provide a collection service. In cases where co-ops are unable or unwilling to provide such a service the Department itself should arrange for collection.

Disinfection of Premises

Based on recommendations by the veterinary profession, the Department has now issued power hoses to District Offices which may be borrowed free of charge by owners of infected herds. These are a great help in the disinfection of premises but there are still many buildings which are impossible to disinfect because of rough walls, loose mortar and other defects. In addition there are careless herdowners who do not appreciate the importance of good hygiene and it is impossible to do much about them, particularly in relation to the storage, disinfection and spreading of manures and slurries. Controls are also needed for slurry spreaders used by contractors. These should be disinfected after each individual farmer's slurry is spread. Some system of checking should be introduced.

The use of better disinfectants should be an ongoing operation. As new products come on the market they should be tried out as a matter of routine by the Department and the Veterinary College. Money for such trials (which would not amount to very much) should be made available in annual budgets.

Financial Contribution from the Farming Sector and Funding of the Scheme Generally

A problem with the eradication scheme over the years has been a lack of continuity of funding by the government. When money is scarce the TB scheme gets a proportional cut in the same way as most other votes. In the previous chapter it was noted that the government had said in 1984 that substantial additional funding was being made available for disease eradication. The White Paper (in which the statement was made) did not say how much the additional funds for eradication should be, but official statements in the press gave the following figures for all disease programmes: £31 million for 1985, £27 million for 1986 and £27 million for 1987. However, in the 1986 budget the suggested figure was cut by £4 million leaving only about £18 million for the TB scheme in that year. This reduction means that testing which cost £11 million in 1985 will have to be reduced by about 40 per cent in 1986 since all the other costs will have to remain the same.

The 1986 funding policy seems to be based on a view that there are large areas of the country free of the disease and that herds in these areas no longer need to be tested on a regular basis. This is a shortsighted policy. Because of our large cattle movement clear areas can very easily become re-infected, as happened many times in the past, and even though it may seem wasteful, there is little option except to continue with annual rounds of testing and the removal of reactors as quickly as possible. If the disease is to be eradicated stop-go policies as regards funding will have to cease. For example, 137 per cent of the national herd was tested in 1985, 61 per cent was tested in 1984 and only 45 per cent in 1982. The present system is no more than a holding operation which stops the disease from reaching an unacceptably high level but will never reduce it to a sufficiently low level. Unfortunately, while the State is the residual funder "stop-go" policies will continue to recur. There must therefore be a change in the funding system. A basic sum must come from the farming community with a matching contribution by the State in the same way as local government rates were matched in the past. If a law to this effect is enacted the government will be compelled to match in some agreed proportion what the farming community pays. These payments should be fixed annually by the Minister for Agriculture on the advice of the Animal Health Council.

The question to be determined then is, what proportion of the funding should the farming community pay, in what form should the payment be made and should those who are free of the disease for some given length of time be exempt from payment? In the previous chapter a view was quoted that levies should be more closely related to outbreaks so as to bring home to herdowners in a positive way the seriousness of the disease problem. This suggestion is based on a thesis that herdowners have it within their power to control the disease on their own holdings if they are forced to do so. Most of the experts would not agree entirely with this view. They admit that herd-owners are very often remiss in their actions and that many are dishonest, but in most cases they have little control over outbreaks of the disease. In a country where there is considerable cattle movement an outbreak can occur on the best managed farm and the whole surrounding area can become contaminated in a matter of weeks. Hence, it seems that the fairest system is to spread the payment over all farms in proportion to final sales of cattle, beef and milk, as is done now. It is true that this system is rather remote from what is happening on the ground but in the ultimate analysis all farmers will benefit from eradication and all should make a contribution to costs. The farmer who is unfortunate enough to have an outbreak is penalised pretty heavily already by having his herd restricted for at least two months and very often for longer periods while, at the same time, receiving very low prices for reactor cattle. It would be unfair to penalise him further unless he is found to be culpably negligent; in that case he should be heavily fined.

The question as to the proportion of the cost which farmers should pay is a difficult one and at the end of the day there is really no objective answer. However, in order to guide policymakers, this question needs to be discussed.

When the disease is eradicated there will be two main beneficiaries, namely:

(1) the herdowners who will have healthier cattle which, along with cattle products, can be marketed without downgrading in price on export markets, and

(2) the government acting *in loco parentis* for the public health and for the public finances which will benefit from enhanced cattle, beef and milk product exports. In equity, therefore, there should be a sharing of costs between these two groups.

However, since farmers are the main beneficiaries they should pay the major portion of the costs. In my opinion a 75 per cent share of the variable costs by herdowners would appear reasonable leaving the government to pay the other 25 per cent and all of the fixed costs which will go on having to be incurred even when the disease is eliminated.

In 1983 the variable costs were £22.3 million to which herdowners contributed £13.0 million or 58 per cent. If the levy were extended to cover cattle slaughtered by butchers a further £1 million would be contributed by herdowners and the ratio would be 63 per cent. To bring this up to 75 per cent the levy on milk would need to be increased to 0.7 pence per gallon and that on cattle to £4.5 per animal. It is recommended that these charges be made forthwith and that they be extended to cattle slaughtered for home consumption if this can be done in a cost effective way. If it cannot, there is no point in making the charge and the other costs should be increased accordingly.

If direct costs increase over time, the levies and the corresponding State contribution should be increased accordingly. Similarly, if costs decrease the levies should be reduced and should be eliminated entirely when the disease is reduced to some agreed level such as, say, 0.5 per cent of herds or .05 per cent of animals. A policy of this kind should create an incentive on the part of farmers to eliminate the disease as quickly as possible and it is felt that in the ultimate analysis they are the only people who can obtain results. In other words, if herdowners are made to "pay the piper" they will ultimately "call the tune".

Transferring the Eradication Scheme to an Executive Office Under a National Manager

Criticisms of the management of the present BTE scheme were put forward in the Conjoint Report of the Veterinary Professions where it was recommended that the operation of the scheme be taken out of the Department of Agriculture and set up as an Executive Office under a National Manager. Many of the criticisms made in the Conjoint Report appear reasonable but as indicated in previous sections of this chapter, it is difficult to do much about them. We must consider, therefore, whether a National Manager operating outside the Department could have a greater degree of success than that being achieved at present.

In favour of the change out of the Department it can be said that a National Manager would be independent of the Minister for Agriculture and could take tough decisions in relation to illegal movement of cattle, bad testing, etc., without fear of political consequences. But it is doubtful if a National Manager could act in a much tougher manner than the present Departmental Manager. He would have his own pressures to contend with. Even with a whole new scheme, the personnel involved would be the same, namely the DVIs and the private practitioners. The latter would be employed to do the same job as they are doing now, on the same holdings and there is no reason to believe that they would change their habits. The Manager might refuse to give testing to some of the more inefficient testers but if he went too far he would have a strike on his hands and he would be back to square one.

In regard to the depopulation of herds the position would be little different from what it is now. The DVIs and the practitioners would have to make these decisions and at the end of the day a lot would depend on the level of the depopulation grant available. There will always be a reluctance to depopulate valuable herds if it means bankrupting the herdowner.

The extent to which holdings can be quarantined, illegal movement of cattle prevented, surveillance at slaughterhouses extended and lorries disinfected, etc., is a function of the amount of money and staff available and there is no reason to believe that the government would be any more generous with an Executive Office than it is at present. Hence the National Manager would have to operate within the same financial constraints as the Department and cut corners for want of cash.

Taking all these points into consideration one has to say that a National Manager would be able to do little more than is being done now. He could make loud noises and threaten vengeance but at the end of the day his teeth would be drawn by all the powerful forces around him, the veterinary profession, the farmers' associations, the Department of Agriculture and the Department of Finance. These bodies would soon cut him down to size.

It could be argued, of course, that the idea of taking the scheme out of the Department should be given a trial, that things cannot be any worse than at present and that there is a chance they could be improved. This suggestion has some appeal until one thinks about the problems and the frictions involved in setting the scheme up as an Executive Office. There would be lengthy negotiations with all the parties concerned; legislation would have to be introduced; the present staff might have to be compensated; the practitioners would probably look for increased testing fees and everybody would want to be on the Board of Directors. It would probably take years to get things sorted out and this would give excuses for reductions in funding and for lack of commitment to the scheme in the meantime. Hence it seems to me that we should stick with what we have and try to improve it. If things do not improve with regular funding, of course, we will have to try something else; public opinion will demand that something drastic be done at that stage.

Strategy Plan

In the above discussion a number of suggestions for improving the scheme have been put forward. But even if all these ideas are implemented there is no guarantee that eradication will be hastened. Everybody involved has become so used to the present system that things will continue to drag on as before unless some unusual policy is adopted. In the White Paper *Building on Reality* the Government said (p. 45)

> The final clearance of bovine TB remains one of the most urgent problems facing agriculture. It is evident that despite substantial cost to the Exchequer little progress towards complete eradication has been achieved over the past few years. Faced with the situation where it is essential to get rid of the disease . . . the Government must be satisfied that funds committed to the programme in future are spent effectively. Since the present arrangements for tackling the disease have not proved effective the Government believes that there must be radical changes in these arrangements. Subject to the introduction of these changes substantial additional funding is being set aside for disease eradication including new special assistance for herd depopulation.

This special assistance has now been made available and a number of the radical changes suggested have been carried out. The latter include:

- Departmental nomination of testers for what it is worth
- payment for testing to be made directly to testers

- payment of reactor grants to be made only if reactors are removed within 10 days, and
- tight official supervision at all marts including, where necessary, control of trading times.

Most of these are important changes, but it is felt that more is needed. All the evidence suggests that at the end of the day there is only one real solution — intensive annual rounds of testing until the disease is deemed to be eradicated. A plan setting a time scale for this event is required, together with an estimate of the annual costs needed to achieve a series of regional targets along the way. Such a trategy will put pressure on the government to enact legislation to provide for a constant level of funding as suggested above and for any other reforms which are deemed to be necessary and feasible.

Special clearance areas may also have to be established, as in the early days of the scheme, but this should be a last resort situation if it is found that targets are not being met. The model with annual targets for different regions is, therefore, of vital importance in order to show where we are going, or if we are going anywhere at all, even with regular funding.

The plan will determine the level of funds required, but a reasonable estimate of variable costs over the coming 4 years is about £28 million per annum at 1985 prices. Nor is there likely to be any saving in overhead costs even with computerisation of the records since there will have to be stricter checks than at present on cattle movement and a general tightening up of the regulations. However, in preparing the plan, a hard look should be taken at the efficiency of administration in the District Offices to see if it can be improved. An examination should be made, preferably by an efficiency expert, to see if the costs here are justified or if, with a re-organisation of effort, we can get more done for the same level of spending.

If and when the plan is put into operation, careful check testing will have to be undertaken to ensure that prescribed targets are being met. This testing will have to be done on a random sample basis as discussed in Chapter 2. The final date set for a defined eradication target should be 1986. If, by the end of 1990 it is found that the target levels set in the plan are not being met, then a re-organisation of the programme will be necessary. In such circumstances the scheme should be set up as an Executive Office and testing taken over entirely by official veterinarians as discussed above under "Nomination of Testers". I am confident, however, that, if we introduce a properly funded scheme for eradication now, this will not be necessary, and that the disease will be reduced to manageable levels by 1990 and virtually eradicated by 1996.

What must be kept in mind, however, is that elimination of the disease (as elimination is normally understood) will not eliminate disease eradication costs. These will have to be incurred indefinitely at about present levels in order to keep tuberculosis, brucellosis and probably other diseases in check. Experience in other countries has shown that there is no way out of this problem and we must live with it. We should learn from our neighbours in Northern Ireland where annual rounds of testing had to be resumed in 1982, some 12 years after it was thought the disease had been eradicated.

REFERENCES

ASHTON, J., A. BUCKWELL, S. ROBSON, 1977. *Veterinary Practice in Ireland, An Economic Study on Behalf of the National Prices Commission*, Dublin: Stationery Office, September, Prl. 7105.

A STRATEGY FOR THE DEVELOPMENT OF IRISH CATTLE AND BEEF INDUSTRY, 1981, Irish Fresh Meat Exporters' Society, Dublin, p. 220.

BADGERS AND T.B. – THE UK EXPERIENCE, *Irish Veterinary News*, December 1985.

BANG, B., 1930. "Experiences from Many Years' Fight Against Bovine Tuberculosis", *The Veterinary Record*, Vol. 10, No. 26.

BOVINE TUBERCULOSIS ERADICATION, 1978. Report of the Department of Agriculture/Department of Finance Study Group, Dublin, February.

BUILDING ON REALITY, 1984. Government White Paper, Stationery Office, Dublin, October.

CHAUSSE, P., 1913. "Des Methodes a Employer Pour Realiser la Tuberculose Experimentale par Inhalation", *Bulletin of the Society for Veterinary Medicine*, Vol. 31, pp. 267-274.

COMMISSION OF THE EUROPEAN COMMUNITIES, 1981. *Commission Report to the Council on the Application of Plans to Accelerate and Intensify the Eradication of Brucellosis, Tuberculosis and Leukosis in Cattle*, Com. 81/611 Final.

CRILLY, J., 1984. Unpublished study in the Library of the Veterinary Research Laboratory, Abbotstown, Dublin.

COLLINS, C.H., and J.H. GRANGE, 1981. "A Review – The Bovine Tubercle Bacillus", *Journal of Applied Bacteriology*, Vol. 55, pp. 13-29.

COLLINS, J.D., 1985. "Tuberculosis in Animals", *Irish Journal of Medical Science*, Vol. 154, Supplement I, May.

CULLEN, R.G., 1982. Bovine TB – the present position in Ireland and what both professions (veterinary and agriculture) can do to accelerate the eradication programme. Proceedings of a Seminar organised by the Irish Veterinary Association and the Agricultural Science Association Liaison Committee, Portlaoise, February.

DISEASE ERADICATION SCHEMES, 1983. Report by Department of Agriculture/Department of Finance Review Group, Dublin, May.

DUNNET, G.M., D.M. JONES, J.P. McINERNEY, 1986. "Badgers and Bovine Tuberculosis", Report to the Rt. Hon. M. Jopling, M.P., and the Rt. Hon. N. Edwards, M.P., London: HMSO, March.

ERADICATION OF TUBERCULOSIS, 1982. Views and Recommendations of the Irish Farmers' Association (March, 1982), the Irish Veterinary Union (April, 1982) and the Irish Veterinary Association (1979) relating to the Recommendations of the Irish Veterinary Association (January).

ERADICATION OF TUBERCULOSIS IN CATTLE, 1984. Conjoint Report of the Irish Veterinary Association, Irish Veterinary Union and the Irish Veterinary Officers' Association.

EVANS, H.T.J., and H.V. THOMPSON, 1980. "Bovine Tuberculosis in Cattle in Great Britain; Eradication of Disease from Cattle and the Role of the Badger (Meles Meles) as a Source of Mycobacterium Bovis for Cattle", *Animal Regulation Studies*, 3, (1980/81), Elsevier Scientific Publishing Co., Amsterdam.

FRANCIS, G., 1958. *Tuberculosis in Animals and Man*, London: Cassel and Company Ltd.

GRANGE, J.M., 1982. "Kocks Tubercle Bacillus, A Centenary Reappraisal", *Zentralblatt für Bakteriologie, Mikrobiologie und Hygiene*, pp. 297-307.

IRISH VETERINARY ASSOCIATION, 1982. Recommendations for the Eradication of Tuberculosis in Cattle, Dublin: 53 Lansdowne Road.

IRISH VETERINARY NEWS, December 1985, Dublin: Tara Street.

IRISH VETERINARY UNION, 1982. Proposals for an Acceleration in the Bovine TB Eradication Scheme, April.

KARDJITO, T., and J.M. GRANGE, 1985. "A Clinical Evaluation of the Diagnostic Usefulness of an Early Dermal Reaction to Tuberculosis: A Failure to Distinguish between Tuberculosis and other Respiratory Diseases", *Tubercle* 66, pp. 129-133.

KERR, W.R., H.G. LAMONT, and J.J. McGIRR, 1946. *Veterinary Record*, Vol. 48, p. 451.

KLEEBERG, H.H., 1960. "The Tuberculin Test", *Journal of the South African Veterinary Medical Association*, Vol. 31, p. 213.

LESSLIE, I.W., and C.N. HEBERT, 1975. *Veterinary Record*, Vol. 96, pp. 338-341.

LESSLIE, I.W., C.N. HEBERT and G.N. FRERISCHS, 1976. *Veterinary Record*, Vol. 98, pp. 170-172.

MacCLANCY, B.N., 1962-63. Reliability of the Single Comparative Intradermal Test, unpublished.

MacCRAE, W.D., 1961. "The Eradication of Bovine Tuberculosis in Great Britain", *Journal of the Royal Agricultural Society of England*, Vol. 122.

MINISTRY OF AGRICULTURE, FISHERIES AND FOOD, Seventh Report, 1983. *Bovine Tuberculosis in Badgers*, London: HMSO.

O'REILLY, L.M., 1969(a). "Accuracy of the Tuberculin Test", (Letter to the Editor), *Irish Veterinary Journal*, Vol. 23, pp. 38-40.

O'REILLY, L.M., 1969(b). "Tuberculosis Eradication — Some Problems of the Post Attestation Era", *Irish Veterinary Journal*, Vol. 23, pp. 140-149.

O'REILLY, L.M., 1982. Bovine Tuberculosis in Calves and Tuberculosis Testing in Calves, Internal Departmental Memorandum.

O'REILLY, L.M., 1985. Tuberculosis in Animals. Report to the Scientific Committee of the International Union Against Tuberculosis, Paris, 30 September-1 October.

O'REILLY, L.M., and B.N. MacCLANCY, 1968. "Tuberculosis — Dual Infections in a Dairy Herd due to Avian and Bovine Type Bacilli", *Irish Veterinary Journal*, Vol. 22, pp. 222-230.

O'REILLY, L.M., and B.N. MacCLANCY, 1975. "A Comparison of the Accuracy of a Human and Bovine Tuberculin PPD for testing Cattle with a Comparative Cervical Test", *Irish Veterinary Journal*, Vol. 29, pp. 63-70.

PATERSON, B., 1959. "Bacteriology of Tuberculosis" in A.W. Stubleforth and I.O. Galloway (eds.), *Infectious Illnesses of Animals; Illnesses of Animals due to Bacteria*, Vol. 2, London: Butterworth.

NATIONAL PLANNING BOARD, April 1984. *Proposal for Plan, 1984-87*, Dublin: Government Publications Sales Office, Prl. 2309.

RITCHIE, J.N., 1959. "Eradication of Bovine Tuberculosis" in A.W. Stubleforth and I.O. Galloway (eds.), *Infectious Illnesses of Animals: Illnesses of Animals due to Bacteria*, Vol. 2, London: Butterworth, pp. 713-736.

ROBERTS, T., 1986. "A Retrospective Assessment of Human Health Protection Benefits from Removal of Tuberculosis Beef", *Journal of Food Protection*, Vol. 49, No. 4, pp. 293-298, April.

ROOK, G.A.W., 1983. "Why Is There No Serodiagnostic Test for Tuberculosis? Will There Be One Soon?", *Paedriatics*, Clinic of India.

SCHWABE, C.N., 1984. *Veterinary Medicine and Human Health*, 3rd Edition, Baltimore: Williams and Wilkins, USA.

SERVING THE COUNTRY BETTER, 1985. A White Paper on the Public Service, Dublin: Stationery Office, Prl. 3262.

STORE CATTLE STUDY GROUP REPORT, 1968. Department of Agriculture and Fisheries, Dublin: Stationery Office, Prl. 297.

SULLIVAN, E.W., 1979. "Tuberculosis in Cattle (1)", *Agriculture in Northern Ireland*, Vol. 53, No. 2.

SULLIVAN, E.W., 1979. "Tuberculosis in Cattle (2)", *Agriculture in Northern Ireland*, Vol. 54, No. 1.

WATCHORN, R.C., 1965. *Bovine Tuberuclosis Eradication Scheme 1954-65*, Department of Agriculture and Fisheries, April.

WILESMITH, J.W., 1983. "Epidemiological Features of Bovine Tuberculosis in Cattle Herds in Great Britain", *Journal of Hygiene*, Vol. 90, pp. 159-176.

LORD ZUCKERMAN, 1980. *Badgers, Cattle and Tuberculosis*, London: Ministry of Agriculture, Fisheries and Food, HMSO, October.

Appendix A

RELIABILITY OF THE TUBERCULIN TEST

In recent years some controversy has arisen in Ireland regarding the reliability of the tuberculin test. At a hearing before the Oireachtais Public Expenditure Committee on the 20 May 1986, Mr L.M. O'Reilly, Senior Research Officer in the Tuberculosis Section of the Department of Agriculture stated that the test, when carried out and interpreted in accordance with the Department's instructions has a specificity of about 99.9 per cent and a sensitivity of about 98 per cent, i.e., an overall reliability of about 99 per cent. At a similar hearing on the 27 May 1986, Professor J.D. Collins of the Veterinary College, UCD, stated that the reliability of the test was only 80-85 per cent and could be as low as 66 per cent in cows. It is difficult to reconcile these two statements. They leave the layperson rather baffled and I can only conclude that the two sides are not talking about the same thing.

Indeed, in a recent article in the *Irish Journal of Medical Science*, Collins (1985) says that:

> in highly infected herds between 2.0 and 9.7 per cent of tuberculosis cattle may be misidentified; however an appraisal of the clinical health of such cattle and reference to their previous testing history would be expected to reduce this figure. Nevertheless, there are other factors such as the often adverse farm conditions under which the tuberculin test is required to be conducted which offer some explanation of the apparent slow progress of eradication to date.

It seems from this that when he speaks of 80-85 per cent reliability Collins is combining the reliability of the test *per se* with the efficacy of its application in practice. O'Reilly, on the other hand, does not take efficacy of application into account. I quote from his document to the Oireachtas Committee:

> The two indices of the reliability of a biological test are *specificity* and *sensitivity*. A test with 100 per cent specificity would ensure

that no disease free animals were classified as reactors.[10] A test with 100 per cent sensitivity would ensure that all diseased animals would react to the test.[11] Therefore, a 100 per cent reliable test would have 100 per cent specificity and 100 per cent sensitivity. Unfortunately, no such test exists. However, this drawback is overcome to a large extent by the inclusion of an inconclusive category in the interpretation keys for both of the tuberculin tests recognised by the EEC (Directive 80/219). The two EEC approved tests are the *single intradermal and the single intradermal comparative tests.*

O'Reilly went on to say:

> In practice it has been found that when there is no inconclusive category in the interpretation key a high sensitivity is only achieved at the cost of a low specificity. The scientific literature indicates that if all animals inconclusive and positive on the standard EEC interpretation were removed the specificity of the comparative test would be as low as 99.1 per cent (Lesslie, *et al.*, 1976). This means that with *exacting careful testing* there would be an overkill of 9,000 disease free cattle per million disease free cattle tested. In 1985 when there were approximately 11 million tests carried out there would have been 122,000 reactors, i.e., a test overkill or wastage of about 99,000 disease free cattle, not to mention the needless restriction of perhaps in excess of 30,000 disease free herds.

In the known infected herds, maintaining the maximum test sensitivity and the early removal of diseased animals are the main priorities. The scientific literature indicates that when inconclusive and positive animals on the standard EEC interpretation are removed as reactors the comparative test in the Irish environment has an overall sensitivity on the basis of skin measurement alone of at least 95 per cent (O'Reilly and MacClancy, 1975; Crilly, 1984) and in the heavily infected herds a sensitivity of 90-98 per cent (Collins, 1985; O'Reilly, 1985). The sensitivity of the comparative test is further increased when a more severe interpretation standard is applied and when further reactors are removed on clinical or epidemiological grounds.

On the basis of O'Reilly's statements and those of the authors which he quotes, it would appear that the test is very reliable under certain conditions, namely:

10. In a test with 90 per cent specificity, 10 per cent of disease free animals would be classed as reactors.
11. In a test with 90 per cent sensitivity, 10 per cent of infected animals would not react to the test.

(a) It is properly carried out.
(b) An inconclusive key is included which allows for removal of such animals from infected herds and for a re-check in 60 days in herds where no conclusive reactors are found.
(c) Clinical and local knowledge are taken into account, i.e., removal of animals in close contact with reactors or animals which the veterinary surgeon, on clinical grounds, might suspect of having the disease.
(d) Animals in close contact with reactors are removed as reactors even though they do not react themselves.

O'Reilly (1969a), however, quotes Kerr, *et al.* (1946) as saying that:

> The single intradermal comparative test was and is primarily designed for use on animals of known history and origin and it was never intended (or held) to be accurate in the case of unknown animals.

In the same article he quotes Kleeberg (1960) as saying that:

> When old cows of unknown origin, possibly from heavily infected herds, are used in experiments to determine the accuracy of the tuberculin test, the number of false negative reactors is certain to be high.

There is also the problem that animals which are negative to the test and in the pre-allergic phase of infection at the time of testing may show up with the disease later on post-mortem examination (O'Reilly, 1985).

Hence, according to O'Reilly's own standards the definition of accuracy is qualified. The history of the population being tested must be known and other information must be made use of for the best results. There is also a problem with old cows which show no reaction to the test but which, nevertheless, are carriers of the disease. O'Reilly also says (1969b) that we must look forward to research work to aid us in obtaining improved means and methods of diagnosis.

But even though the test is reliable (when carried out under the conditions specified above) there are problems with its application in practice. As stated in Chapter 1 and by Collins (1985), the conditions under which the test has to be applied and the carelessness of some of the testers are probably the crucial factors in identifying reactors or otherwise. It is for these reasons that a reliable blood test is sought which can be applied in the laboratory under ideal conditions, particularly to blood samples of suspected carriers of the disease which do not show reaction to the skin test. Unfortunately, worldwide research over the last 80 years has not succeeded in developing such a test. Nor does there seem to be such a test round the corner as many commentators would have us believe.

Rook (1983) discussing human tuberculosis has said that:

> an enormous amount of time and money has been spent in efforts to improve the diagnostic value of antibody assays using crude antigens but these all fail because of the high levels of antibody to cross-reacting organisms present in all normal sera, and the relatively low levels found in sera of some severely ill patients. Subsequent attempts to overcome this problem by isolating species specific antigens of M tuberculosis have proved unexpectedly difficult.

He went on to say:

> now, however, there is a real possibility that monoclonal antibodies will allow development of an inhibition assay for antibody which is specific for M tuberculosis or even capture assays for myco bacterial antigen in CSF serum or urine. Nevertheless, there are still serious theoretical problems.

This was written in 1983, yet in 1985 Kardjito and Grange (1985) refer to disillusionment among research workers with the results of serological tests. They state that in many instances blood tests "that showed promise when initially evaluated with sera from known cases of tuberculosis and from healthy control subjects failed miserably when applied in routine clinical practice".

Appendix B

REACTOR COMPENSATION – RATES OF GRANT (JUNE, 1986)

TB	Non-Pedigree	Pedigree
Cows and in-calf heifers	£225	£285
Other cattle under 182 kgs.	£210	£250
Other cattle 182 kgs. and over	£85	£125

Brucellosis		
Cows and in-calf heifers	£175	£225
Other cattle under 182 kgs.	£170	£205
Other cattle 182 kgs. and over	£75	£115

Latent Carriers

An *ex gratia* payment of £100 per head is payable on the removal of certain non-reacting animals considered to be latent carriers of infection, up to a limit of three animals per herd.

De-population Fund Scheme

The scheme provides additional compensation for herdowners whose herds have to be de-populated because of serious infection with TB or Brucellosis.

Payment is at the rate of £100 per qualifying animal subject, in the case of TB, to a maximum payment of £10,000.[12]

Qualifying animals are cows, in-calf heifers, bulls and also other cattle which kill out at under 182 kgs. They include those in the herd at the time of de-population and other animals in the categories mentioned which were removed as reactors in the previous 12 months.

Stock Replacement Scheme

Payment is at the rate of £40 – or £60 where the herdowner leaves dairying – in respect of each animal on which a payment under the De-population Fund Scheme is made, up to a maximum of £4,000 and £6,000 respectively.[13]

---

12. Maximum payments refer to TB.
13. No limit in case of Brucellosis.

Appendix C

THE EPIDEMIOLOGY OF TUBERCULOSIS CONTRASTED WITH THAT OF BRUCELLOSIS

(1) For tuberculosis the infective dose is very low. Chausse (1913) has shown that not more than five bacilli, and probably only one, can produce a lesion in the lung of a bovine animal. He showed on the basis of experiments that direct droplet infection and the inhalation of infective dust are both important sources of infection. In the case of brucellosis the infective dose is quite high. The challenge dose is 15 million organisms.

(2) There is no immunity based on age or sex for tuberculosis whereas only sexually mature animals show symptoms of brucellosis.

(3) Almost all tuberculosis infected cattle are open cases (spreaders of the disease). Complete healing of lung lesions which often takes place in man seldom occurs in cattle. Attempts in the past to identify so-called "open" and closed cases of tuberculosis by clinical and bacteriological methods have failed and the only method found effective was the slaughter of all tuberculosis positive animals (Bang's Method), (Bang, 1930). Only pregnant animals shed the brucellosis organism and they do this only for a short time after parturition or abortion. The organism may, however, be shed in milk.

(4) Transmission of tuberculosis occurs 24 hours a day throughout the year and lateral spread often occurs along river banks and across fences. Spread is much more rapid when animals are under stressful conditions, e.g., when travelling, in pregnancy, outlying in winter and when on poor rations. Well-fed animals have reasonably good resistance. Transmission of brucellosis is limited mainly to the calving season when the foetal membranes are expelled and for a few weeks afterwards.

(5) Tuberculosis is an insidious disease. There is very often no clinical evidence to alert the herdowner. Brucellosis is not an insidious disease. When an abortion outbreak occurs the farmer is very much aware of the loss of calves and lowered milk yields.

(6) A wide range of animals may act as a reservoir for M. bovis infection, e.g., badgers, red deer, pet dogs, cats and goats. No other animal has been

shown to directly transmit brucellosis infection to cattle.

(7) Tubercle bacilli are very resistant to environmental conditions. The following survival times have been recorded for M. bovis: 1 year in faecal pats, 5 months in liquid manure and slurry, 7 months in water, 6 to 8 months in dried sputum and 7 weeks on grass. The bacilli are very resistant to disinfectants. Immersion for 1 hour in 5 per cent phenol is necessary to kill both M. bovis and M. tuberculosis. Brucellosis organisms are readily killed by disinfectants.

(8) There is no laboratory screening test available to diagnose tuberculosis and because of the nature of the disease no such test is likely to be found in the near future (see Appendix A). There is, therefore, no absolutely effective control over the official testing of cattle for bovine tuberculosis. Reliance has to be placed on each veterinarian to carry out the test in accordance with instructions. In addition there is the possibility that the herdowner may attempt to influence the tester in the interpretation of the test, particularly when it comes to declaring "in contact" animals as reactors when they are negative to the test. There is an effective blood test for diagnosing brucellosis which is carried out in a laboratory without pressure from herdowners.

(9) There is no effective vaccine available for tuberculosis.   BCG has given disappointing results when used on cattle. There is an approved vaccine available for brucellosis.

Books:

Economic Growth in Ireland: The Experience Since 1947
Kieran A. Kennedy and Brendan Dowling
Irish Economic Policy: A Review of Major Issues
Staff Members of ESRI (eds. B. R. Dowling and J. Durkan)
The Irish Economy and Society in the 1980s (Papers presented at ESRI Twenty-first Anniversary Conference)
Staff Members of ESRI
The Economic and Social State of The Nation
J. F. Meenan, M. P. Fogarty, J. Kavanagh and L. Ryan
The Irish Economy: Policy and Performance 1972-1981
P. Bacon, J. Durkan and J. O'Leary
Employment and Unemployment Policy for Ireland
Staff Members of ESRI (eds., Denis Conniffe and Kieran A. Kennedy)
Public Social Expenditure – Value for Money? (Papers presented at a Conference, 20 November 1984)
Medium-Term Outlook: 1986–1990. No. 1
Peter Bacon

Policy Research Series:

1. *Regional Policy and the Full-Employment Target* M. Ross and B. Walsh
2. *Energy Demand in Ireland, Projections and Policy Issues* S. Scott
3. *Some Issues in the Methodology of Attitude Research* E. E. Davis *et al.*
4. *Land Drainage Policy in Ireland* Richard Bruton and Frank J. Convery
5. *Recent Trends in Youth Unemployment* J. J. Sexton
6. *The Economic Consequences of European Union. A Symposium on Some Policy Aspects*
D. Scott, J. Bradley, J. D. FitzGerald and M. Ross
7. *The National Debt and Economic Policy in the Medium Term* John D. FitzGerald

Broadsheet Series:

1. *Dental Services in Ireland* P. R. Kaim-Caudle
2. *We Can Stop Rising Prices* M. P. Fogarty
3. *Pharmaceutical Services in Ireland* P. R. Kaim-Caudle
assisted by Annette O'Toole and Kathleen O'Donoghue
4. *Ophthalmic Services in Ireland* P. R. Kaim-Caudle
assisted by Kathleen O'Donoghue and Annette O'Toole
5. *Irish Pensions Schemes, 1969* P. R. Kaim-Caudle and J. G. Byrne
assisted by Annette O'Toole
6. *The Social Science Percentage Nuisance* R. C. Geary
7. *Poverty in Ireland: Research Priorities* Brendan M. Walsh
8. *Irish Entrepreneurs Speak for Themselves* M. P. Fogarty
9. *Marital Desertion in Dublin: An Exploratory Study* Kathleen O'Higgins
10. *Equalization of Opportunity in Ireland: Statistical Aspects*
R. C. Geary and F. S. Ó Muircheartaigh
11. *Public Social Expenditure in Ireland* Finola Kennedy
12. *Problems in Economic Planning and Policy Formation in Ireland, 1958–1974*
Desmond Norton
13. *Crisis in the Cattle Industry* R. O'Connor and P. Keogh
14. *A Study of Schemes for the Relief of Unemployment in Ireland*
R. C. Geary and M. Dempsey
with Appendix E. Costa
15. *Dublin Simon Community, 1971-1976: An Exploration* Ian Hart

16. *Aspects of the Swedish Economy and their Relevance to Ireland*
                    Robert O'Connor, Eoin O'Malley and Anthony Foley
17. *The Irish Housing System: A Critical Overview*
                                        T. J. Baker and L. M. O'Brien
18. *The Irish Itinerants: Some Demographic, Economic and Educational Aspects*
                                        M. Dempsey and R. C. Geary
19. *A Study of Industrial Workers' Co-operatives*
                                    Robert O'Connor and Philip Kelly
20. *Drinking in Ireland: A Review of Trends in Alcohol Consumption, Alcohol Related Problems and Policies towards Alcohol*   Brendan M. Walsh
21. *A Review of the Common Agricultural Policy and the Implications of Modified Systems for Ireland*   R. O'Connor, C. Guiomard and J. Devereux
22. *Policy Aspects of Land-Use Planning in Ireland*
                                    Frank J. Convery and A. Allan Schmid
23. *Issues in Adoption in Ireland*   Harold J. Abramson

Geary Lecture Series:
1. *A Simple Approach to Macro-economic Dynamics* (1967)   R. G. D. Allen
2. *Computers, Statistics and Planning-Systems or Chaos?* (1968)   F. G. Foster
3. *The Dual Career Family* (1970)   Rhona and Robert Rapoport
4. *The Psychosonomics of Rising Prices* (1971)   H. A. Turner
5. *An Interdisciplinary Approach to the Measurement of Utility or Welfare* (1972)
                                                    J. Tinbergen
6. *Econometric Forecasting from Lagged Relationships* (1973)   M. G. Kendall
7. *Towards a New Objectivity* (1974)   Alvin W. Gouldner
8. *Structural Analysis in Sociology* (1975)   Robert K. Merton
9. *British Economic Growth 1951-1973: Success or Failure?* (1976)
                                                R. C. O. Matthews
10. *Official Statisticians and Econometricians in the Present Day World* (1977)
                                                E. Malinvaud
11. *Political and Institutional Economics* (1978)   Gunnar Myrdal
12. *The Dilemmas of a Socialist Economy: The Hungarian Experience* (1979)
                                                János Kornai
13. *The Story of a Social Experiment and Some Reflections* (1980)
                                            Robert M. Solow
14. *Modernisation and Religion* (1981)   P. L. Berger
15. *Poor, Relatively Speaking* (1983)   Amartya K. Sen
16. *Towards More Rational Decisions on Criminals* (1984)   Daniel Glaser
17. *An Economic Analysis of the Family* (1985)   Gary S. Becker

General Research Series:
1. *The Ownership of Personal Property in Ireland*   Edward Nevin
2. *Short-Term Economic Forecasting and its Application in Ireland*   Alfred Kuehn
3. *The Irish Tariff and The E.E.C.: A Factual Survey*   Edward Nevin
4. *Demand Relationships for Ireland*   C. E. V. Leser
5. *Local Government Finance in Ireland: A Preliminary Survey*   David Walker
6. *Prospects of the Irish Economy in 1962*   Alfred Kuehn
7. *The Irish Woollen and Worsted Industry, 1946-59: A Study in StatisticalMethod*
                                                R. C. Geary

ESRI PUBLICATIONS

8. *The Allocation of Public Funds for Social Development* David Walker
9. *The Irish Price Level: A Comparative Study* Edward Nevin
10. *Inland Transport in Ireland: A Factual Study* D. J. Reynolds
11. *Public Debt and Economic Development* Edward Nevin
12. *Wages in Ireland, 1946-62* Edward Nevin
13. *Road Transport: The Problems and Prospects in Ireland* D. J. Reynolds
14. *Imports and Economic Growth in Ireland, 1947-61* C. E. V. Leser
15. *The Irish Economy in 1962 and 1963* C. E. V. Leser
16. *Irish County Incomes in 1960* E. A. Attwood and R. C. Geary
17. *The Capital Stock of Irish Industry* Edward Nevin
18. *Local Government Finance and County Incomes* David Walker
19. *Industrial Relations in Ireland: The Background* David O'Mahony
20. *Social Security in Ireland and Western Europe* P. R. Kaim-Caudle
21. *The Irish Economy in 1963 and 1964* C. E. V. Leser
22. *The Cost Structure of Irish Industry 1950-60* Edward Nevin
23. *A Further Analysis of Irish Household Budget Data, 1951-52* C. E. V. Leser
24. *Economic Aspects of Industrial Relations* David O'Mahony
25. *Phychological Barriers to Economic Achievement* P. Pentony
26. *Seasonality in Irish Economic Statistics* C. E. V. Leser
27. *The Irish Economy in 1964 and 1965* C. E. V. Leser
28. *Housing in Ireland: Some Economic Aspects* P. R. Kaim-Caudle
29. *A Statistical Study of Wages, Prices and Employment in the Irish Manufacturing Sector* C. St. J. O'Herlihy
30. *Fuel and Power in Ireland: Part I. Energy Consumption in 1970* J. L. Booth
31. *Determinants of Wage Inflation in Ireland* Keith Cowling
32. *Regional Employment Patterns in the Republic of Ireland* T. J. Baker
33. *The Irish Economy in 1966* The Staff of The Economic Research Institute
34. *Fuel and Power in Ireland: Part II. Electricity and Turf* J. L. Booth
35. *Fuel and Power in Ireland: Part III. International and Temporal Aspects of Energy Consumption* J. L. Booth
36. *Institutional Aspects of Commercial and Central Banking in Ireland* John Hein
37. *Fuel and Power in Ireland: Part IV. Sources and Uses of Energy* J. L. Booth
38. *A Study of Imports* C. E. V. Leser
39. *The Irish Economy in 1967* The Staff of The Economic and Social Research Institute
40. *Some Aspects of Price Inflation in Ireland* R. C. Geary and J. L. Pratschke
41. *A Medium Term Planning Model for Ireland* David Simpson
42. *Some Irish Population Problems Reconsidered* Brendan M. Walsh
43. *The Irish Brain Drain* Richard Lynn
44. *A Method of Estimating the Stock of Capital in Northern Ireland Manufacturing Industry: Limitations and Applications* C. W. Jefferson
45. *An Input-Output Analysis of the Agricultural Sector of the Irish Economy in 1964* R. O'Connor with M. Breslin
46. *The Implications for Cattle Producers of Seasonal Price Fluctuations* R. O'Connor
47. *Transport in the Developing Economy of Ireland* John Blackwell
48. *Social Status and Inter-Generational Social Mobility in Dublin* Bertram Hutchinson

ESRI PUBLICATIONS

49. *Personal Incomes by County, 1965*   Miceal Ross
50. *Income-Expenditure Relations in Ireland, 1965-1966*   John L. Pratschke
51. *Costs and Prices in Transportable Goods Industries*
                                          W. Black, J. V. Simpson, D. G. Slattery
52. *Certain Aspects of Non-Agricultural Unemployment in Ireland*
                                                      R. C. Geary and J. G. Hughes
53. *A Study of Demand Elasticities for Irish Imports*   Dermot McAleese
54. *Internal Migration in Ireland*   R. C. Geary and J. G. Hughes
    with Appendix   C. J. Gillman
55. *Religion and Demographic Behaviour in Ireland*   B. M. Walsh
    with Appendix   R. C. Geary and J. G. Hughes
56. *Views on Pay Increases, Fringe Benefits and Low Pay*
                                          H. Behrend, A. Knowles and J. Davies
57. *Views on Income Differentials and the Economic Situation*
                                          H. Behrend, A. Knowles and J. Davies
58. *Computers in Ireland*   F. G. Foster
59. *National Differences in Anxiety*   Richard Lynn
60. *Capital Statistics for Irish Manufacturing Industry*   C. W. Jefferson
61. *Rural Household Budget – Feasibility Study*   Sile Sheehy and R. O'Connor
62. *Effective Tariffs and the Structure of Industrial Protection in Ireland*
                                                                  Dermot McAleese
63. *Methodology of Personal Income Estimation by County*   Miceal Ross
64. *Further Data on County Incomes in the Sixties*   Miceal Ross
65. *The Functional Distribution of Income in Ireland, 1938-70*   J. G. Hughes
66. *Irish Input-Output Structures, 1964 and 1968*   E. W. Henry
67. *Social Status in Dublin: Marriage, Mobility and First Employment*
                                                              Bertram Hutchinson
68. *An Economic Evaluation of Irish Salmon Fishing, I: The Visiting Anglers*
                                                      R. O'Connor and B. J. Whelan
69. *Women and Employment in Ireland: Results of a National Survey*
                                          Brendan M. Walsh assisted by Annette O'Toole
70. *Irish Manufactured Imports from the UK in the Sixties: The Effects of AIFTA*
                                                  Dermot McAleese and John Martin
71. *Alphabetical Voting: A Study of the 1973 General Election in the Republic of Ireland*
                                          Christopher Robson and Brendan M. Walsh
72. *A Study of the Irish Cattle and Beef Industries*
                                  Terence J. Baker, Robert O'Connor and Rory Dunne
73. *Regional Employment Patterns in Northern Ireland*
                                          William Black and Clifford W. Jefferson
74. *Irish Full Employment Structures, 1968 and 1975*   E. W. Henry
75. *An Economic Evaluation of Irish Salmon Fishing II: The Irish Anglers*
                                          R. O'Connor, B. J. Whelan and A. McCashin
76. *Factors Relating to Reconviction among Young Dublin Probationers*   Ian Hart
77. *The Structure of Unemployment in Ireland, 1954-1972*   Brendan M. Walsh
78. *An Economic Evaluation of Irish Salmon Fishing, III: The Commercial Fishermen*
                                          B. J. Whelan, R. O'Connor and A. McCashin
79. *Wage Inflation and Wage Leadership*
                                          W. E. J. McCarthy, J. F. O'Brien and V. G. Dowd

80. *An Econometric Study of the Irish Postal Service*   Peter Neary

81. *Employment Relationships in Irish Counties*

Terence J. Baker and Miceal Ross

82. *Irish Input-Output Income Multipliers 1964 and 1968*

J. R. Copeland and E. W. Henry

83. *A Study of the Structure and Determinants of the Behavioural Component of Social Attitudes in Ireland*   E. E. Davis

84. *Economic Aspects of Local Authority Expenditure and Finance*

J. R. Copeland and Brendan M. Walsh

85. *Population Growth and other Statistics of Middle-sized Irish Towns*

D. Curtin, R. C. Geary, T. A. Grimes and B. Menton

86. *The Income Sensitivity of the Personal Income Tax Base in Ireland, 1947-1972*

Brendan R. Dowling

87. *Traditional Families? From Culturally Prescribed to Negotiated Roles in Farm Families*   Damian F. Hannan and Louise Katsiaouni

88. *An Irish Personality Differential: A Technique for Measuring Affective and Cognitive Dimensions of Attitudes Towards Persons*   E. E. Davis and Mary O'Neill

89. *Redundancy and Re-Employment in Ireland*

Brendan J. Whelan and Brendan M. Walsh

90. *A National Model for Fuel Allocation – A Prototype*   E. W. Henry and S. Scott

91. *A Linear Programming Model for Irish Agriculture*

Robert O'Connor, Miceal Ross and Michael Behan

92. *Irish Educational Expenditures – Past, Present and Future*   A. Dale Tussing

93. *The Working and Living Conditions of Civil Service Typists*

Nóirín O'Broin and Gillian Farren

94. *Irish Public Debt*   Richard Bruton

95. *Output and Employment in the Irish Food Industry to 1990*

A. D. O'Rourke and T. P. McStay

96. *Displacement and Development: Class, Kinship and Social Change in Irish Rural Communities*   Damian F. Hannan

97. *Attitudes in the Republic of Ireland Relevant to the Northern Problem: Vol. I: Descriptive Analysis and Some Comparisons with Attitudes in Northern Ireland and Great Britain*   E. E. Davis and R. Sinnott

98. *Internal Migration Flows in Ireland and their Determinants*

J. G. Hughes and B. M. Walsh

99. *Irish Input-Output Structures, 1976*   E. W. Henry

100. *Development of the Irish Sea Fishing Industry and its Regional Implications*

R. O'Connor, J. A. Crutchfield, B. J. Whelan and K. E. Mellon

101. *Employment Conditions and Job Satisfaction: The Distribution, Perception and Evaluation of Job Rewards*   Christopher T. Whelan

102. *Crime in the Republic of Ireland: Statistical Trends and Their Interpretation*

David B. Rottman

103. *Measure of the Capital Stock in the Irish Manufacturing Sector, 1945-1973*

R. N. Vaughan

104. *A Study of National Wage Agreements in Ireland*   James F. O'Brien

105. *Socio-Economic Impact of the Construction of the ESB Power Station at Moneypoint, Co. Clare*   R. O'Connor, J. A. Crutchfield and B. J. Whelan

ESRI PUBLICATIONS

106. *The Financing of Third-level Education*   A. C. Barlow
107. *An Input-Output Analysis of New Industry in Ireland in 1976*   E. W. Henry
108. *Social Insurance and Absence from Work in Ireland*   Gerard Hughes
109. *The Distribution of Income in the Republic of Ireland: A Study in Social Class and Family-Cycle Inequalities*
David B. Rottman, Damian F. Hannan and Niamh Hardiman,
Miriam M. Wiley
110 *The Economic and Social Circumstances of the Elderly in Ireland*
B. J. Whelan and R. N. Vaughan
111. *Worker Priorities, Trust in Management and Prospects for Workers' Participation*
Christopher T. Whelan
112. *The Impact of Energy Prices on the Irish Economy during 1973-1981*
E. W. Henry
113. *Schooling and Sex Roles: Sex Differences in Subject Provision and Student Choice in Irish Post-Primary Schools*
D. Hannan, R. Breen and B. Murray, D. Watson, N. Hardiman,
K. O'Higgins
114. *Energy Crops, Forestry and Regional Development in Ireland*
Frank J. Convery and Kathleen Dripchak
115. *Aggregate Supply, Aggregate Demand and Income Distribution in Ireland: A Macro-sectoral Analysis*   John Bradley and Connell Fanning
116. *Social Mobility in the Republic of Ireland: A Comparative Perspective*
Christopher T. Whelan and Brendan J. Whelan
117. *Attitudes towards Poverty and Related Social Issues in Ireland*
E. E. Davis, Joel W. Grube and Mark Morgan
118. *A Study of New House Prices in Ireland in the Seventies*
Ian J. Irvine
119. *Education and the Labour Market: Work and Unemployment Among Recent Cohorts of Irish School Leavers*
Richard Breen
120. *Payroll Tax Incidence, the Direct Tax Burden and the Rate of Return on State Pension Contributions in Ireland*   Gerard Hughes
121. *Crime Victimisation in the Republic of Ireland*
Richard Breen and David B. Rottman
122. *Medium-term Analysis of Fiscal Policy in Ireland: A Macroeconometric Study of the Period 1967-1980*
John Bradley, Connell Fanning, Canice Prendergast and Mark Wynne
123. *The Irish Wealth Tax A Case Study in Economics and Politics*
Cedric Sandford and Oliver Morrissey
124. *Aspects of Freight Transport in Ireland*   Jack Short
125. *Small-Scale Manufacturing Industry in Ireland*
Kieran A. Kennedy and Tom Healy (assisted by J. Bergin, T. Callan and
P. McNutt)
126. *Irish Medical Care Resources: An Economic Analysis*   A. Dale Tussing
127. *Employment in the Public Domain in Recent Decades*   Miceal Ross
128. *Multisector Modelling of the Irish Economy With Speical Reference to Employment Projections*   E. W. Henry

129. *Subject Availability and Student Performance in the Senior Cycle of Irish Post-Primary Schools*   Richard Breen

130. *A Statistical Analysis of the Irish Electoral Register and its Use for Population Estimation*   Gary Keogh and Brendan J. Whelan

131. *The Population Structure and Living Circumstances of Irish Travellers: Results from the 1981 Census of Traveller Families*

David B. Rottman, A. Dale Tussing and Miriam M. Wiley

132. *Smoking, Drinking and Other Drug Use Among Dublin Post-Primary School Pupils*

Joel W. Grube and Mark Morgan